Alternative Therapies

Alternative Therapies

Swati Bhagat PT

BPT
Diploma in Yoga Therapy
PGD in Preventive and Promotive Health Care
Diploma in Acupuncture
Diploma in Food and Nutrition

Incharge Knee Club
Sancheti Institute of
Orthopaedics and Rehabilitation
16, Shivaji Nagar, Pune

JAYPEE BROTHERS
MEDICAL PUBLISHERS (P) LTD
New Delhi

Published by

Jitendar P Vij
Jaypee Brothers Medical Publishers (P) Ltd
EMCA House, 23/23B Ansari Road, Daryaganj
New Delhi 110 002, India
Phones: 23272143, 23272703, 23282021, 23245672, 23245683
Fax: 011-23276490 e-mail: jpmedpub@del2.vsnl.net.in
Visit our website: http://www.jpbros.20m.com

Branches

- 202 Batavia Chambers, 8 Kumara Kruppa Road, Kumara Park East
  Bangalore 560 001, Phones: 2285971, 2382956 Tele Fax: 2281761
  e-mail: jaypeebc@bgl.vsnl.net.in

- 282 IIIrd Floor, Khaleel Shirazi Estate, Fountain Plaza
  Pantheon Road, **Chennai** 600 008, Phone: 28262665 Fax: 28262331
  e-mail: jpmedpub@md3.vsnl.net.in

- 4-2-1067/1-3, Ist Floor, Balaji Building, Ramkote Cross Road
  Hyderabad 500 095, Phones: 55610020, 24758498   Fax: 24758499
  e-mail: jpmedpub@rediffmail.com

- 1A Indian Mirror Street, Wellington Square
  Kolkata 700 013, Phone: 22451926 Fax: 22456075
  e-mail: jpbcal@cal.vsnl.net.in

- 106 Amit Industrial Estate, 61 Dr SS Rao Road, Near MGM Hospital
  Parel, **Mumbai** 400 012, Phones: 24124863, 24104532 Fax: 24160828
  e-mail: jpmedpub@bom7.vsnl.net.in

Alternative Therapies

This book has been published in good faith that the material provided by author is original. Every effort is made to ensure accuracy of material, but the publisher, printer and author will not be held responsible for any inadvertent error(s). In case of any dispute, all legal matters to be settled under Delhi jurisdiction only.

First Edition: **2004**

ISBN   81-8061-220-1

Typeset at   JPBMP typesetting unit
Printed at   Replika Press Pvt. Ltd.

My Pranams
To
Maa   Santhoshi
Without Her Blessings
This Book Would Not
Have Been Possible

Preface

I assembled this book with the hope of making the study a little easier.

I have included a number of subjects from the core of yoga, which deals its implementation in different conditions. A significant portion of the book has been allotted to Naturopathy, Acupuncture, Magnetotherapy and Nutrition.

It is my belief that all sections including Stress Management should be known for the treatment of various conditions.

Any suggestion and advice for the improvement in the form and contents of this book would be welcome to the author.

Swatimano;@rediffmail.com
gv_swati@yahoo.com

Swati Bhagat PT

Contents

Section 1
Yoga

Section 2

Stress Management

Section 3
Naturopathy

Section 4
Magnetotherapy

Section 5
Acupuncture

Section 6

Nutrition

SECTION 1
YOGA

chapter one

What is Yoga?

Yoga is the union of individual 'Self', 'Jeevatma', with the universal self, 'Paramatma'. It is the communion of the human soul with the divinity. The essence of our existence is our individual principle of Consciousness or the simple meaning of 'Yog' is union.

Yoga is the integration and harmony between thoughts, words, and deeds or integration between head, heart, and hands.

Patanjali, writer of the classical yogic text, *The Yogasutras,* defines yoga as—"Complete control over the different patterns or modifications of consciousness."

WHY YOGA?

Our actions in the outside world cause us pain or pleasure. These waves of pain and pleasure in our heart, 'Chitta', cause upheavals of emotions.
They are:
1. Kama (infatuation)
2. Krodha (Anger)
3. Lobha (Greed)
4. Moha (Lust)
5. Mada (Pride)
6. Matsara (Malice).

The scriptures explain these six emotions as the main enemies of man. These emotions consume energy of man. In order to minimize this waste of energy, 'Rishis', the seers of yore, discovered the discipline of yoga.

Three 'Gunas'—(a) Tamas, (b) Rajas and (c) Sattwa control our activities in this world—which are the agents of Cosmic 'Prakriti' and 'Purusha'. They pervade our bodily existence and control our activities.

Tamas Guna

Tamas means inertia or a static state. It also means ignorance or darkness. In natural sleep, one neither experiences one's own existence, nor witnesses the state of sleep. The Consciousness is totally under the influence of 'Tamo Guna' in sleep. After natural sleep, 'tamoguna' offers the entry in sattwa and rajo guna activity and offers virtue of serenity. However, in wakeful state, the continued 'tamoguna' gives inertia, rest, and laziness.

Rajas Guna

Rajas guna helps to maintain the beat of physical activity. In spiritual practice, 'rajasic' activity is used to pierce and penetrate towards the core of the being. Asana, Pranayama practice, is rajasic activity. This activity purifies the rajo guna. The scriptures proclaim that the pure rajo guna is essential to approach Sattwa guna.

Sattwa Guna

Sattwa means illumination, the illumination of intelligence. Under the influence of Sattwa Guna, the activity is done with more attention to the core of the being, that is attention to mind, intelligence, and consciousness. This activity gives knowledge, tranquility, and joy. The spiritual practice is possible only in Sattwa activity.

We have to cross all these three Gunas' activities to reach and to live in Purusha, the pure consciousness.

THE EIGHT STAGES OF YOGA

The eight stages of yoga are—Yama, Niyama, Asana, Pranayama, Pratyahara, Dharana, Dhyana, and Samadhi; the first step, of yoga is *YAMA*.

Yama

Yama includes universal moral and ethical commandments. They help the practitioner to identify the same 'self' as in others, as in himself.

There are five YAMAS –

- **Ahimsa**—The simple meaning of Ahimsa is not to hurt anybody. Not to inflict physical or mental pain to anybody, not to inflict any pain or violence upon one's body—all these come under the sphere of Ahimsa.
- **Satya**—The simple meaning of Satya is 'reality'.
- **Asatya**—The simple meaning of Asatya is not to steal. The practitioner controls his desires and reduces his wants.
- **Brahmacharya**—The simple meaning of Brahmacharya is to lead a controlled sex life, even as a householder living in a society. Righteousness and virtue should guard the demand. Raw sense enjoyment must not be the motive.
- **Aparigraha**—The meaning of Aparigraha is not to collect. We should have only as much as is necessary.

Niyam

The second component or step of yoga is Niyam. They are five in number. Niyams are the rules of self-purification.

- **Shauch (purity)**—The simple meaning of shauch is cleanliness or purity. Purity is of two types, external and internal. External purity is clean habits, cleanliness of self and surroundings. Internal purity is purification of mind. It is achieved by uprooting the 'six enemies in the path of self-realization. The six enemies are passion (kama), anger (krodha), greed (lobha), infatuation (moha), pride (mada), and malice (matsara).

- **Santosh (contentment)**—The simple meaning of Santosh is to be content with whatever you get. This reduces desire.
- **Tap (austerity)**—To be efficient, tolerant and to be victorious over difficulties, is the simple meaning of Tapas. In society, Tap does not mean to do meditation in a cave, but to develop physical and mental tolerance; to keep one's senses controlled, to keep the mind controlled, not to be disturbed in hunger, thirst, cold, or heat, but to tolerate them and to remain contented in these situations and to adapt oneself to the environment is called 'Tap.'
- **Swadhyaya (self-study)**—The easy meaning of Swadhyaya is 'study'. The study of scriptures is done to educate oneself in the knowledge of the 'truth' and the 'self'. We should do Swadhyaya according to our capacity and availability of time; age and time should be taken into consideration for Swadhyaya.
- **Ishwarapranidhana (worship of God)**—The surrender of all our actions to the Lord and abiding entirely in 'His will' is Ishwarapranidhana.

Practice of Yama, Niyama reduces the ego desires and causes dominance of 'Sattwa Guna' in the aspirant's 'Chitta'. This gives stability and concentration to the 'Chitta'.

Asana

Asana means taking a posture, by placing hands, feet, and body trunk in a particular posture. They are innumerable, catering to various physical and mental needs of the person. During Asana practice, the practitioner is in 'Annamaya Kasha'. The 'consciousness' is involved in the actions of the body and in the sensation invoked by the actions. The activity is done with the idea of purifying the individual's body and mind. Asana caters to the various needs of the musculoskeletal, digestive, circulatory, respiratory, hormonal, glandular, nervous, and other systems of the body. By practicing Asana, the practitioner overcomes the physical disabilities, mental disturbances, and the gates of the spiritual practice open to him. The freshness and lightness has to be experienced in both the body and the mind. The mind has to be alert, knowledgeable, and honest to pick up which and how much Asana should be done.

Pranayama

Pranayama is a conscious inhalation, retention, and exhalation of breath. There are two words in Pranayama, Prana and Ayama. The meaning of the Sanskrit word Prana is life force, oxygen and breath. Ayama means to lengthen, to spread, to control, and to retain. Thus Pranayama means 'lengthening, controlling, and retaining of life force'.

Breathing in, breathing out, and controlling breathing, the three processes together is known as Pranayama.

Rechaka—The process of exhaling or breathing out.

Puraka—The process of inhaling or breathing in.

Kumbhaka—The process of retaining breathe.

There are two Kumbhakas:

1. **Internal Kumbhaka**—The action of retaining breathe after inhaling.
2. **External Kumbhaka**—The action of not breathing in after breathing out.

Advantages

The practice of Pranayama makes the lungs flexible and strong. The body gets sufficient oxygen. Blood is purified and has a very good effect on the brain. Pranayam practice stimulates the physico-physiological body, biological body, and psychological body of the practitioner to give correct balance to his body and the mind.

It also cures constipation, strengthens the intestines and the nervous system.

SOME GUIDELINES TO BE FOLLOWED BEFORE PRACTICING PRANAYAMA

- It should be done in an open space, such as garden, terrace, while sitting on a blanket, carpet, or mat.
- The place should be clean and quiet, and it should not be done in strong breeze or where the air is foul or has a bad smell or smoke.
- Pranayama should not be done after a heavy meal.
- Before practicing, one should go to the toilet and also take bath.
- Clothing should be light and loose.
- For practicing Pranayama, the best asana is the Padmasana. If not possible, it can also be done in the Sukhasana or Siddhasana.
- The waist, back, and neck should remain erect during the procedure.

Pratyahara

Pratyahara means 'gathering towards'. The mind received sensory impulses from the outside world and the body and also from extra-sensory perceptions from the self. In Pratyahara, the extrovert senses are quietened down, and they are turned inwards. With the inward-turned eyes and ears, one experienced optical and auditory extrasensory perceptions. The practitioner starts believing in the system only when he gets the glimpses of optical or auditory extrasensory perceptions.

Dharana

When 'Chitta' the mind, intelligence, consciousness is confined and limited to a certain place in the body, it is Dharana. The mind should be made to think of one point in the heart or between the two eyebrows on the forehead.

Dhayana

When Dharana continues for a long time, it becomes 'Dhyana'—meditation. In Dhayana, there is no movement in the body and the mind intelligence unit. Meditation cannot be taught. It is a subjective experience. It is an indescribable state that has to be experienced. It releases all tension. In meditation, the flow of energy is continuous and stable. The awareness of space and time is lost.

Samadhi

When the uninterrupted flow of the individual's awareness gets absorbed in the object of 'meditation', his 'consciousness' loses its identity and becomes one with the object. The merging of the individual's consciousness in the object of meditation is a total consummation called 'Samadhi'.

chapter two

Yogic Physiology

At the time of the creation of the gross universe, the five great beings are in 'subtle bodies', that is, in the mind or in the 'consciousness unit'. The 'gross bodies' of the five great beings are formed by combination with one another. All gross bodies come into existence from all pervading 'space'—Aakasha. The space 'Aakasha' symbolizes 'Paramatma'. The cosmic 'Prakriti Shakti' is symbolized by air 'Vayu'. It is the root cause of all movement. After this, fire, water, and earth are created.

These elements combine with one another in a certain ratio—that is half of itself plus one-eighth of each of the other four. This process is called 'Panchikarana'. When the gross bodies are formed.

Aakasha—space manifests itself as sound.
Vayu—air manifests itself as sound and touch.
Tej—fire manifests itself as sound, touch, and form.
Aap—water manifests itself as sound, touch, form, and taste.
Prithvi—earth manifests itself as sound, touch, form, taste, and smell.

Thus each succeeding element has a specific quality of its own. These specific qualities of the 'five great elements' carry knowledge about that element. This knowledge is received in our body by the sense organs.

Thus—
- Ears give knowledge of 'sound'—the space element.
- Skin gives knowledge of 'touch'—the air element.
- Eyes give knowledge of 'form'—the fire element.
- Tongue gives knowledge of 'taste'—the water element.
- Nose gives knowledge of 'smell'—the earth element.

THE BODY EXPLAINED IN TERMS OF THE FIVE GREAT BEINGS

The five vital airs—*Pancha Prana*—are the energies of the principle of consciousness of the five great beings. 'Pancha Prana' controls the working of all the body cells and the different physiological system of the body. 'Prana' is the most important vital air. The other four vital airs interact with 'Prana' individually or in a group to bring about the physiological function.

The Earth Principle

All solid particles of the body—minerals, proteins, carbohydrates, and fats are grouped under the earth principle. The earth gives boundary, size, and shape to the various cells and the tissues of the body. The absolute materialization in the 'Apana' energy of the earth in the body is the 'bone formation'. Bones give size, shape, and support to the body.

'Apana' energy is stored in the lower pelvis around rectum and anus. The movement of the pelvis, buttocks, thighs, legs, and feet are controlled by 'Apana' energy. The excreta, the urine, the semen, fetus, are thrown out of the body under the influence of the 'Apana' energy. 'Apana' energy plays an essential role in respiration.

The Water Principle

All the 'liquids' in the body belong to the water. Intracellular fluids, extracellular fluids, tissue lymph fluids, and blood are all water. Body water is a vehicle for nutrients, foods, gases, oxygen, carbon dioxide, and body waste products. The respiratory waves of inspiration and expiration are the subtle water forms.

'Prana' the energy of consciousness of water principle is essential for each and every physiological function of the body. 'Prana' is mainly stored in the head and chest regions. The functions of the mind—intelligence, brain, heart, lungs, five action organs, and five sensory organs are controlled by 'prana'. The urinary bladder function is the 'sole' of water element functioning in the body.

The Fire Principle

In our body, muscle tissue represents the fire principle. During muscle contractions, muscle carbohydrates are broken down to release the heat and other energies. These energies are utilized for effecting joint movements and for nourishing bones—*Asthi-Poshan*. The process of converting stored food into energy and energy into stored food is called metabolism.

Samana energy is the energy of the principle of consciousness of 'Fire'. This energy controls digestion, absorption, and assimilation of food. Samana energy is also responsible for undigested excreta from food.

The Air Principle

All 'airs'—gases—in the body represent the matter forms of 'Udana' energy. Air that carries MAIN PRANA is the Prana Vayu or Oxygen. Main Prana is the 'soul' of Vayu Tattwa in the body. Air principle is responsible for all types of movement in the body.

'Udana' energy is stored in the chest in the region of the heart. This energy circulates around the nose, wind pipe, throat, and neck. Memory, effort, determination, will power, zest for life, texture and the color of the skin, and speech are the functions controlled by the 'Udana' energy in the body.

The Space Principle

The space 'Akasha' pervades the whole of the body. All spaces in the body—intracellular spaces, extracellular spaces, joint spaces, the space in the chest cavity, and the abdominal cavity—

represent matter form of the 'Vyana' energy. The space in the abdominal cavity is the soul of 'Akasha Tatwa' in the body.

'Vyana' is the energy that remains in the body, especially in the abdomen, chest, and in the heart at the end of expiration and before the next inspiration. 'Vyana' energy is a state between 'Prana' and 'Apana'. Sound production is the absolute function of 'Vyana' energy.

The movements of the trunk and limbs: expansion and deflation. Stretching and shortening is the function of 'Vyana'. The opening and closing of the eyelids is also the function of Vyana.

chapter three

Anatomy and Physiology for the Yoga Learner

The following description of the human anatomy and physiology illustrates the basic principles about the functioning of the body.

The material is discussed under the following headings:

1. A note on the functional organization of the human body and control of the 'Internal Environment'.
2. The Earth Principle—'Prithvi Tatwa'—consisting of skin and musculoskeletal structures.
3. The Water Principle—'Aap Tatwa'—consisting of the circulatory and respiratory system.
4. The Fire Principle—'Tej Tatwa'—consisting of metabolism and the endocrine system.
5. The Air Principle—'Vayu Tatwa'—consisting of the nervous system.
6. The Space Principle—'Aakasha Tatwa'—consisting of body spaces.

FUNCTIONAL ORGANIZATION OF THE HUMAN BODY AND CONTROL OF THE INTERNAL ENVIRONMENT

The human body is made up of millions of cells. The basic living unit of the human body is a cell. Each organ is an aggregate of many different cells.

Each cell is a discrete unit enclosed by a membrane. The cell membrane envelops the living aqueous (water) called cytoplasm or protoplasm. Cytoplasm contains one or more nuclei. The cytoplasm of the cell consists chemically of large and small organic molecules and inorganic ions in an aqueous solution. The nucleus, which contains genes and nucleic acids DNA and RNA, is responsible for hereditary instructions. The nucleus, according to Yogic science, is the 'mind and intelligence' center for the cell.

Extracellular fluid lies outside the cell filling the space in between the cell (intracellular) space. Extracellular fluid is in constant motion. It contains and supplies all the ions, nutrients, and oxygen needed by the cells for cellular life. The end toxic product such as water, carbon dioxide, etc. are discharged in the extracellular fluid. Thus, the extracellular fluid essentially forms the 'SAME' internal environment for all the different cells.

The cells, live, grow, reproduce, and perform their specific functions only when they have sufficient oxygen, glucose, different ions, amino acids, and fatty acids.

The principal substances from which cells extract energy are oxygen, water, and food. This energy is the life force of the living cells. This energy is extracted from nature.

Medical science tries to correlate this energy with the element manifestations of nature's resources like oxygen, water, food, heat, etc. Yogic science, on the other hand, goes beyond this and relates to the life force 'Pranic Shakti' with the 'Cosmic Source'. According to Yogic science, oxygen (Vayu), is the vehicle for cosmic 'Pranic Shakti'. Food means trapped and stored Sun energy. The minerals and the solids of food means the Earth.

Essentially all the organs and the various systems of the body perform functions that help to maintain the condition of the extracellular fluid constant.

In very broad terms, various systems of the body work as follows:

1. *Lung and blood circulation*—provides oxygen to the extracellular fluid for use by the cells and remove carbon dioxide that is formed in the cells.
2. *Kidneys*—maintain constant mineral concentration in the extracellular fluid. They also regulate the water mass of the body.
3. *Heart*—pumps blood to the capillaries from where there is a free exchange between the extracellular fluid and the blood. Blood carries oxygen, carbon dioxide, nutrients, waste products, and hormones, therefore, a carriage vehicle.
4. *Gastrointestinal system*—collects, digests, and releases nutrients to the blood.
5. *Immune system*—is involved with the resistance of the body to infection. Our body is normally exposed to bacteria, viruses, fungi, and parasites. Many of these agents are capable of invading deeper tissues. They can cause serious disruption in the functioning of the cells.

    The human body has the ability to resist almost all types of organisms or toxins that tend to damage the cells, the tissues, or the organs. This capacity of the body to resist is called immunity.

    This is achieved in two different ways.

    A. Destroying the invading agents by a process known as 'Phagocytosis', engulfing the foreign material, destroying it, and digesting the debris and the foreign body, e.g.—white blood cells (WBC macrophages).
    B. Destruction by formation of antibodies and sensitizing the lymphocytes, one or both of which may destroy the invader. This is called the Acquired Immune Response, e.g.—Lymphocyte.

6. *Hormonal system (Endocrine)*—Hormones are chemical substances secreted in the blood by the endocrine glands. They are transported to the extracellular fluid to reach all parts of the body to help in regulation of cellular function. Hormonal system mainly regulates the metabolic functions of the cell.
7. *Nervous system*—The nervous system is the supreme control of all body functions. In general, it regulates mainly muscular and secretary activities of the voluntary and involuntary systems of the body. It also governs the hormonal system.

The nervous system is important to know because it is the 'matter representation' of the 'subtle' and the 'causal' body of the individual. Thus, the nervous system is the seat of the mind—intelligence—ego and the consciousness of the individual. So it is a must to know the basic details of the nervous system.

The functional unit of the nervous system is a nerve cell with its process. The whole structure is known as Neuron. Nerve cell conducts impulses in only one direction.

Dendrites convey impulses to the nerve cell. There are many dendrites to each neuron. They are sensory in nature (Dayanendriya).

Axons convey impulses away from the nerve cell. The nerve cell usually has only one axon. It is motor in function (Karmendriya). Pathways are established within the nervous system by connection between the neurons via the dendrites.

Cell bodies with similar functions show a great tendency to group themselves into aggregates known as ganglions, nuclei, or nerve centers. The fibers from such aggregations of cell bodies tend to run together in bundles. These bundles, when they are inside the brain and spinal cord are known as tracts. When they lie outside the brain or spinal cord, they are known as peripheral nerves.

Broadly, the nervous system is divided into two parts:

I. The Somatic (Voluntary) Nervous System.

II. The Autonomic (Involuntary) Nervous System.

The Somatic Nervous System—(Soma = Body)

In general, the somatic nervous system supplies the outer body and is under the control of conscious will.

It is further divided into two parts:

1. The Central Nervous System—contains the Brain and the Spinal Cord, containing the tracts.
2. The Peripheral Nervous System—consists of the peripheral nerves. These are called 'Cranial' nerves if they exit out of brain, or 'Spinal' nerves if they exit out of spinal cord. Both cranial and spinal nerves supply sensory and motor nerves to the body.

The Autonomic Nervous System (Automatic = Involuntary, (Auto = Self, Nomos = Law)).

This control all the involuntary functions of the body over which we have no conscious control, such as circulation, digestion, formation of urine, beating of the heart and so forth.

There are three types of muscle in the body.

i. **The skeletal muscle**: We can move this muscle at will. It is under the control of somatic nervous system.

ii. **The non-skeletal muscle**: It is also known as smooth muscle. This lines the wall of the digestive organs such as the stomach and intestine, and is also present in the respiratory and urogenital system. It is not under the control of our will or our conscious mind.

iii. **The highly striated muscle of the heart**: This is again not under control of our will.

The automatic nervous system is concerned with innervation of the non-skeletal and the heart muscle as well as the many glands of the body such as the salivary glands, sweat glands and the hormonal glands like thyroid, adrenals, pituitary and so forth. It also supplies the digestive and respiratory passage.

It is further subdivided into two parts:

1. The sympathetic nervous system ('Surya Nadi' to yoga science).
2. The parasympathetic nervous system ('Chandra Nadi' to yoga science).

Both system give branches and supply to the involuntary organs mentioned above. Their effects in such cases are antagonistic (opposite) to each other.

In general, the effects are as follows—

1. **Parasympathetic system**: The parasympathetic system tends to produce a well sustained vegetative tranquil state (slow pulse, glands secreting, hollow, viscera (organs) undergoing peristalisis with sphincters relaxed.

2. **Sympathetic system**: The sympathetic system produces the opposite effects so necessary in a state of emergency reaction (Rapid pulse, high blood pressure, salivary and digestive glands not secreting, sphincters closed). These changes result in increased work of the cardiovascular system and a raised metabolism. Sympathetic stimulation is aptly described as a 'Fight or Flight' response as opposed to the vegetative tranquil state of Parasympathetic stimulation.

Stimulation of the sympathetic nervous system takes place when limbs, bodywall, and the eyeball muscles work against the gravity or in an angry excited state of mind.

This whole-integrated working of the nervous system is arranged according to a definite plan of sensory to connect pathways to motor pathways, through connections called Synapses between the neurons.

The central nervous system consists of the brain and the spinal cord.

The brain consists of the Cerebral hemispheres, the base of brain, the brain stem, and the cerebellum.

The brain stem—This is a part that connects the brain to the spinal cord.

The cerebellum is that part of the brain, situated on the back of the brain stem.

The two halves of the brain, taken together with the spinal cord, we have 5 levels in the nervous system, where the functions are executed.

1. **The spinal cord function**—The spinal cord conduct the signals from the periphery of the body to the brain and from the brain back to the body via the various tracts.

   Spinal reflex action—It is important to note that the reflex actions (actions not controlled by conscious thought process) also occurs at the spinal cord level. To mention a few, these include reflexes that control respiration and heart actions, walking movements, stiffening of the legs to support the body against gravity, local blood vessels regulation, gastrointestinal movements, digestive activity, activity of the adrenal glands.

2. **The brain stem**—This connects the spinal cord to the brain. Nerve cells of many life controlling systems such as heart, circulation, respiration is located here.

   Various chemicals called neurotransmitters are released here in response to incoming stimuli. These are capable of quickly altering the autonomic functions according to the need.

3. **The cerebellum**—The cerebellum is concerned with the planning of motor activity. It also monitors and makes corrective adjustments in the motor activities elicited by other parts of the nervous system. It deals with equilibrium and balance of the body. Cerebellum is vital to control very rapid muscular activities like running, typing, talking.

4. **The base of the brain**—It is very important to know the function because it is the automatic control center, hormonal master glands (like pituitary), emotional, behavioral centers for gross skeletal muscle (motor) actions are situated in this area. The chief centers are also located in this area.

5. **The cerebral hemispheres**—The two halves of the brain are the seat of intelligence. They act as a storehouse for sensory memories. They initiate voluntary motor actions.

Mode of Action of the Nervous System

Most activities of the nervous system is initiated by sensory experiences or their memories. The somatic nervous system receives special sensations from the environment such as smell, taste, sight, touch and hearing.

The motor response of the sensory information depends on the interpretive capacity of the individual. The interpretive capacity or the intelligence is always colored or influenced by the egoistic attitude, desires or the emotions of the individual. Depending on this interpretation, the motor response will either be tranquil or agitated either parasympathetic (tranquil) or sympathetic (agitated). The response of the skeletal muscles, the involuntary muscle (both smooth and heart muscle) and the glands will depend on which sections of the autonomic nervous system is stimulated, parasympathetic or sympathetic.

During and after the motor activity, a reactionary second wave of sensory impulses is carried to the central nervous system. The reactionary sensory waves again start a new motor activity, so on and so forth.

Somatic sensory receptors carry information from the entire body surface, as well as from the deeper structures like muscles and bones via spinal cord to the cerebral cortex.

Visceral sensory nervous system carries information about the nutrition, oxygenation of tissues, viscosity and PH of the blood.

There is other control systems in the body. Some operate within the organs to control the individual parts of the organ, other operates throughout the entire body to control the inter-relationship between the organs. For example, the respiratory system, operating in the association with the nervous system, regulates the concentration of carbon dioxide in the extracellular fluid.

The most intricate of these control systems is the genetic control system. This operates within the cell to control all life processes and the intracellular functions.

Thus essentially, all the organs and the tissues of the body perform functions that help to maintain the extracellular fluid or internal environment of the body constant at all times.

These functions are controlled at cellular level or at whole individual level by the nervous system of the body.

Yogic science goes beyond medical science. The latter recognizes and stops at nervous control of cellular function. Yogic science, on the other hand, accepts cellular mind, intelligence, consciousness and the concept of all pervading 'PRANA—The Vital Force'. It also believes that the vital life force can be carried to different sites in the body through the unifying role of individual consciousness.

chapter four

Some Important Guidelines and Cautions for Practice of Asanas

1. The best time to practice yoga is early morning before breakfast, or with a very light snacks.
   Any time it should be done in empty stomach, ie. two hours after a light meal or four hours after a meal.
2. Evacuate your bowel and bladder.
3. Preferably bathe before and after practising asanas. It refreshes body and mind.
4. Yogasanas should preferably be done in empty stomach, Vajrasan is the only asan which can be done after a meal
5. Practice in a warm, quite, clean, and airy place. There should be proper ventilation. Do not perform asanas on bare floor or uneven place. Blanket or mat can be used.
6. Dress should be loose and comfortable.
7. Ladies should not do asanas during the advance stage of pregnancy or menstruation.
8. Do not practice asanas after being out in the hot sun for several hours.
9. Start the session with 5 minutes of toning up exercises to loosen the joints and the body.
10. Breathing should be done through the nose only.
11. Standing asanas should be done first, followed by sitting, lying and inverted asanas, backward bends, twists, and forward bend. End the session with 5-10 minutes of savasana.
12. Avoid jerky movements while doing asanas. Any asanas should not be completed with a jerk. It might produce pain, and harm the body.
13. Practice asanas with full concentration and awareness of the bodypart.
14. Exale during all forward bending movements in which the chest and abdomen is being compressed, and inhale during all backward bending movements in which the chest or abdomen is being expanded. Breath normally while maintaining the pose.
15. In the beginning any asanas should be done for a shorter duration (2 or 3 minute), this time can be gradually increased, and the final posture can be maintained as long as possible without any physical or mental strain.
16. Coming out of the final pose must be done by retracing the steps of going into the final pose of asanas.
17. Do not force your body to achieve final pose.
18. If practising in a group do not compete with others.
19. If you have any medical problem, consult your doctor as well as inform your yoga teacher.

20. Asanas can be done after modification by taking proper guidance from an expert and experienced yoga teacher in serious cardiovascular, respiratory and orthopedic disorders.

21. Person with severe myopia, and those suffering from hypertension, glaucoma , detachment of retina, discharging ears and cervical spondylitis must avoid inverted asanas.

22. All the asanas can be practised during the first three months of pregnancy. All the standing pose or forward bending asanas may be done with mild movement, no extra pressure should be given on the abdomen. Baddha konasana and Upavistha konasana may be practised throughout pregnancy as it helps to strengthen the pelvic floor muscle and also helps to reduce labor pain. Pranayama without retention may be practised throughout the pregnancy, as regular deep breathing will help during labor.

23. A warm bath before and 15 minutes after the session will help people who have severe arthritis.

24. Positive effects will be observed after 3 months of regular and sincere practice.

25. Pranayama should be done early in the morning. Persons with heart or lung problems or in case of insomnia, poor memory and concentration should not do Kumbhaka or stoppage of breath.

Meditation should be done in the early morning or at night just before retiring.

chapter five

Asanas that Helps to Cure Disease and Symptoms

Disease and Symptoms	Group of Asanas	Name of Asanas
Obesity	Standing asanas, Forward bending, Backward bending and twist.	Garudasana, Parighasana, Gomukhasana, Ardhachandrasana, Pawanmuktasana, Ekapada Rajakapotasana, Urdhva Dhanurasana, Ardha Matsyendrasana, Bharadvajasana.
Arthritis, Backache, and Spondylitis	Stress reducing asanas, Backward bend asanas and twist	Supta Baddha Konasana, Garudasana, Anantasana, Supta Virasana, Salbhasana, Bhujangasana, Ustrasana, Urdha Mukha Svanasana, Urdhva Dhanurasana, Dhanurasana.
Asthma, Bronchitis, Chronic lung obstruction, Chronic cough, Bronchiectasis, cold	Forward bend, Backward bend, Stress reducing asanas, Nadi Sodhana, Pranayama without 'Khumbka'	Supta Baddha Konasana, Supta Virasana, Adhomukha Svanasana, Urdha Mukha Svanasana, Bhujangasana, Janu Sirsasana, Urdha Dhanurasana, Pascimottanasana, Yoga Mudra, Ujjayi Pranayama, Nadi Sodhana Pranayama.
Diabetes	Forward bend, Backward bend, twist, Stress reducing asanas	Supta Virasana, Adhomukha Virasana, Pawanmuktasana, Halasana, Bhujangasana, Bharadvajasana, Janu Sirsasana, Pascimottanasana, Nadi Sodhana Pranayama.

Contd...

Contd...

Disease and Symptoms	Group of Asanas	Name of Asanas
High Blood Pressure	Forward bend with head resting on support, Stress reducing asanas, Nadi Sodhana Pranayama without retention of breath and meditation	Adhomukha Virasana, Supta Baddha Konasana, Janu Sirsasana, Savasana, Nadi Sodhana Pranayama, Sanmukhi Mudra, Dhyana.
Low Blood Pressure	Forward bends, Backward bends, Inverted asanas, Nadi Sodhana Pranayama without retention of breath	Uttanasana, Parsvottanasana Salamba Sarvangasana, Adhomukha Svanasana, Prasarita Padottanasana, Salamba Sirsasana, Bhujangasana, Urdha Mukha Svanasana, Ustrasana, Dhanurasana.
Cerebral conditions– Insomania, Migraine, Poor concentration and memory	Inverted asanas, Stress reducing asanas, Ujjayi and Nadi Sodhana Pranayama without retention of breath and meditation	Uttanasana, Supta Baddha Konasana, Salamba Sarvangasana, Prasarita Padottanasana, Sirsasana, Savasasana, Sanmukhi Mudra.
Dyspepsia, Constipation, Peptic ulcers	Forward bend, Stress reducing asanas, Nadi Sodhana Pranayama	Virasana, Adhomukha Virasana, Supta Baddha Konasana, Supta Virasana, Pawanmuktasana, Ardhachandrasana, Janu Sirasasana, Pascimottanasana, Yoga Mudra, Ujjayi Pranayama, Nadi Sodhana Pranayama.
Hyperacidity	Forward bend with head resting on support, Stress relieving asanas	Virasana, Adhomukha Virasana, Supta Baddha Konasana, Makarasana, Anantasana, Janu Sirsasana, Pascimottanasana, Savasana, Nadi Sodhana Pranayama.

Contd...

Contd...

Disease and Symptoms	Group of Asanas	Name of Asanas
Menstrual disorders, Dsymenorrhoea, Irregular periods	Forward bend, Stress reducing asanas, Ujjayi and Nadi Sodhana, Pranayama, avoid asanas during periods	Baddha Konasana, Virasana, Adhomukha Virasana, Supta Baddha Konasana, Supta Virasana, Prasarita Padottanasana, Anantasana, Janu Sirsasana, Pascimottanasana

TADASANA (MOUNTAIN POSE)

Tada means mountain, Sama means upright straight, Sthiti means standing still, steadiness.

Technique

- Stand erect with feet together.
- Keep the abdomen in, chest forward, spine stretched up and shoulder braced backwards.
- Maintain the pose and breathe normally.
- Ideally in *Tadasana*, the arms are stretched out over the head.

Advantages

- Helps to correct posture.
- Straightens the spine.
- Strengthens the muscle of abdomen and extremities.
- Broadens shoulders and chest.
- Reduces fat around thigh and abdomen.
- Strengthens joints of lower extremities.
- Tones abdominal organs.

Indications

- Postural deformities of spine.
- Faulty postures and gait.
- Weakness of legs.
- Drooping shoulders.
- Visceroptosis.
- Narrow chest.

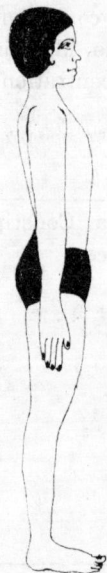

Figure 5.1: Tadasana

VRKSASANA (TREE POSE)

Vrksa means a tree.

Technique

- Stand in *Tadasana*.
- Take right leg up and place foot on the left thigh, as high as possible, toes pointing down.
- Keep left leg straight, with knee locked.
- Balance and keep hands in prayer position.
- Inhale and raise both hands up straight over the head, palms facing each other.
- Maintain the pose and breathe normally.
- Exhale and return to original pose.

Advantages

- Tones leg muscle.
- Improves balance and co-ordination.
- Straightens the spine.
- Strengthens the knee and loosen the hip joint.
- Strengthens the shoulders.

Indications

- Postural deformities of spine.
- Weakness of legs and shoulders.
- Arthritis of joints of upper and lower extremities.

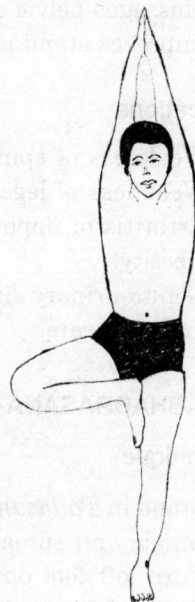

Figure 5.2: Vrksasana

UTKATASANA (POWERFUL POSE)

Utkata means powerful, fierce, uneven. This asana is like sitting on an imaginary chair.

Technique

- Stand in *Tadasana*.
- Inhale and stretch arms straight up, palms facing each other in prayer position.
- Exhale, bend the knee and lower the trunk till the thighs are parallel to the floor.
- Keep back straight, chest as far back as possible and feet flat on the ground.
- Maintain posture and breathe normally.
- Inhale and resume erect posture.
- Exhale and bring arms down to normal position.

Advantages

- Removes stiffness in the shoulders.
- Strengthens muscles of upper and lower extremities, abdomen and diaphragm.
- Tones the spine.
- Strengthens ankle, knee, hip and shoulder joint.
- Reduces fat in thighs and calves.
- Massages pelvic organs.
- Improves stamina.

Indications

- Weakness of spine.
- Weakness of legs and abdominal muscles.
- Arthritis of upper and lower extremity.
- Obesity.
- Genito-urinary disorders of urinary bladder, uterus, ovaries, testes and prostrate.

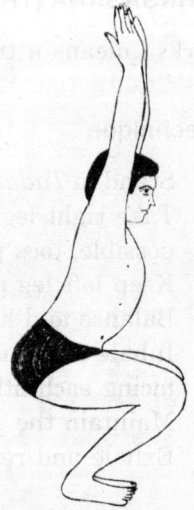

Figure 5.3: Utkatasana

VIRABHADRASANA-II (VIRABHADRASANA POSE)

Technique

- Stand in *Tadasana*.
- Inhale and spread leg 4 feet apart and keep arms parallel to floor.
- Turn left foot out 90 degree and right foot in 30 degree.
- Bend left leg to right angle, allowing the torso to descend vertically downwards at the same spot with navel pointing forward.
- Look towards the left and gaze at the fingers of the left hand.
- Maintain the pose and breathe normally.
- Inhale and return to the original position by retracing the steps in the reverse order.
- Repeat pose on opposite side.

Advantages

- Strengthens leg, thigh, abdominal and neck muscles.
- Tones abdominal and pelvic organs.
- Removes stiffness from all joints.
- Reduces fat around arm and thighs.
- Elongates and strengthens the spine.
- Improves stamina.

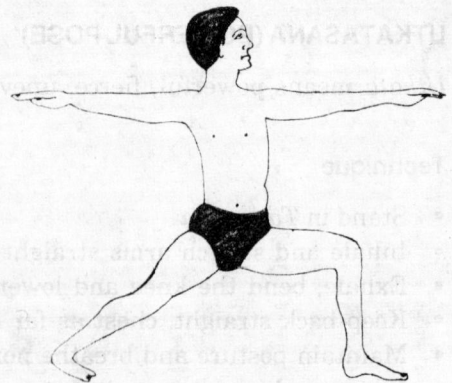

Figure 5.4: Virabhadrasana-II

Indications

- Weakness of arms and legs.
- Disorders of abdominal and pelvic organ.
- Arthritis.
- Obesity involving arm, thighs or abdomen.
- Stiffness of spine.

UTTHITA TRIKONASANA (EXTENDED TRIANGLE POSE)

Technique

- Stands in *Tadasana*.
- Inhale and spread legs 3 or 4 feet apart.
- Raise arm to a horizontal level and keep them parallel to the floor.
- Turn left foot out 90 degree and right foot in 30 degree.
- Exhale and bend trunk towards the left, allows left palm to rest on the floor, close to and behind the left heel.
- Raise right arm up in line with the opposite shoulder.
- Look towards the right thumb.
- Maintain the pose and breathe normally.
- Inhale and return to original pose retracing the steps in a reverse order. Repeat the pose on the opposite side.

Advantages

- Tones up leg muscle.
- Removes stiffness in the legs and hips.
- Tones abdominal and respiratory organs.
- Strengthens spine and the neck.
- Tones muscles of the side of chest, abdomen and leg.
- Strengthens ankle, knee and shoulder joints.
- Improves stamina and balance.

Indications

- Gastro-intestinal disorders of stomach liver, spleen and intestines.
- Respiratory disorders, chronic bronchitis and asthma.
- Backache and spondylitis.
- Weakness of legs.
- Weak angles and knee joints.
- Broad waist and thighs.

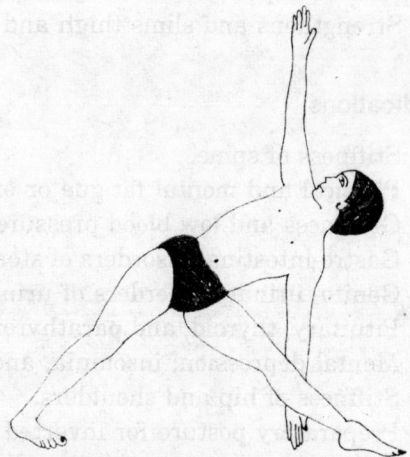

Figure 5.5: Utthita Trikonasana

UTTANASANA (SPINE STRETCHING POSE)

UT is a particle indicating intensity, 'tan' means to stretch, extend. In this asana the spine is given a deliberate and an intense stretch.

Technique

- Stand in *Tadasana*, keeping the knees tight.
- Inhale, extend arms up along the sides and face palms forward.
- Exhale, bend trunk and extend arms forward and downward and allow hands to touch floor or place palm on floor.
- Exhale and allow trunk to move closer to legs and the head to sink downwards and rest forehead on the shins.
- Keep both legs erect and perpendicular to floor and neck totally relaxed.
- Maintain the pose and breathe normally.
- Inhale and return to original pose.

Advantages

- Stretches spine.
- Improve blood flow to head and neck.
- Improves blood flow to hypothalamus, pituitary, pineal, thyroid, parathyroid, and thymus glands.
- Massages abdominal and pelvic organs.
- Soothes nerves and calms mind.
- Tones gonads.
- Loosens hip and shoulder joints.
- Strengthens and slims thigh and calf.

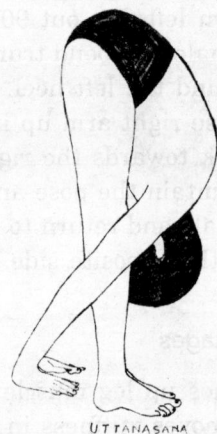

Figure 5.6: Uttanasana

Indications

- Stiffness of spine.
- Physical and mental fatigue or exhaustion.
- Giddiness and low blood pressure.
- Gastro-intestinal disorders of stomach, intestine, liver, gall bladder, spleen and pancreas.
- Genito- urinary disorders of urinary bladder, uterus, prostate.
- Pituitary, thyroid, and parathyroid disorders.
- Mental depression, insomnia, and lack of concentration.
- Stiffness of hip and shoulders.
- Preparatory posture for inverted asana.

VIRABHADRASANA-I (VIRBHADRASANA)

Technique

- Stand in *Tadasana*.
- Inhale, spread legs 4 to 4.5 feet apart, raising both arms to horizontal level.
- Inhale and raise both arms vertically, palms facing each other.
- Exhale and twist to the left with left foot turning 90 degree and right foot 30 degree, so that trunk and navel face towards the left.
- Exhale and bend left knee to a right angle and extend head and neck upward to look up.
- Keep right leg completely stretched and outer border of foot and heel in contact with floor.
- Maintain the pose and breathe normally.
- Exhale and return to original position by retracing the steps in the reverse order.
- Repeat the same for opposite leg.

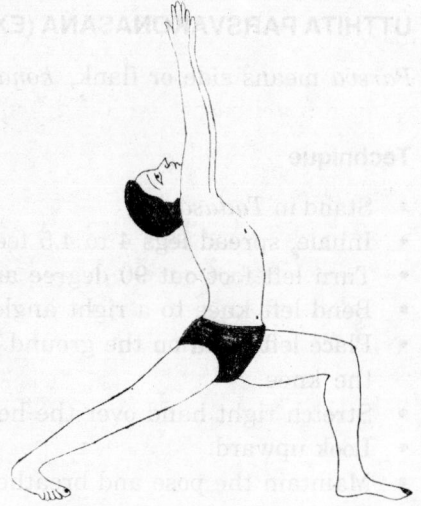

Figure 5.7: Virabhadrasana-I

Advantages

- Tones the spine
- Tones larynx, chest, abdominal and pelvic organs.
- Strengthens leg muscles and improves stamina.
- Helps to strengthen all joints.
- Reduces fat around waist.
- Stimulate thyroid gland.

Indications

- Cervical spondylitis.
- Voice disorders.
- Asthma and bronchitis.
- Digestive and pelvic organ disorders.
- Menstrual disorders.
- Weakness of legs.
- Arthritis.
- Drooping shoulder.
- Fat around waist, hip and thigh.
- Thyroid disorder.

UTTHITA PARSVAKONASANA (EXTENDED LATERAL ANGLE POSE)

Parsva means side or flank, *'kona'* means angle.

Technique

- Stand in *Tadasana*.
- Inhale, spread legs 4 to 4.5 feet apart, spread both arms horizontally parallel to floor.
- Turn left foot out 90 degree and right foot in 30 degree.
- Bend left knee to a right angle, allowing trunk to descend vertically
- Place left hand on the ground close to outer border of left heel and left armpit touching the knee.
- Stretch right hand over the head with palm facing down.
- Look upward.
- Maintain the pose and breathe normally.
- Inhale and return to original position.
- Repeat the same for opposite side.

Advantages

- Stretches and strengthens the spine.
- Stretches lateral chest muscles, and waist along with upper and lower extremities.
- Tones muscle of neck.
- Tones heart, abdominal organs and gonads.
- Strengthens all joints of upper and lower extremities.
- Reduces obesity around waist, arms and legs.
- Increases stamina.

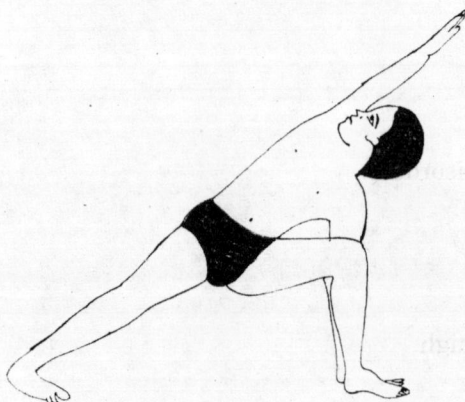

Figure 5.7: Utthita parsvakonasana

Indications

- Spondylitis.
- Weakness of upper and lower extremities.
- Arthritis.
- Obesity of abdomen, arms or hips.
- Gastro-intestinal, respiratory and sexual disorders.
- General weakness.

GARUDASANA (EAGLE POSE)

Technique

- Stand in *Tadasana*.
- Bend right knee slightly, and place left thigh over the right.
- Twist left calf around the right, so that left big toe hooks around the inner side of the right calf.
- Cross right elbow over the left, twist left forearm around the right, so that palm comes in proximity and face each other.
- Raise arms to shoulder level and straighten and elongate the back.
- Straighten right knee as much as possible.
- Maintain the pose and breathe normally.
- Exhale and return to original pose.
- Repeat pose with the opposite leg and arm in the front.

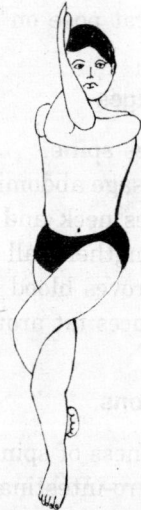

Advantages

- Loosen joints of both extremities.
- Tones and strengthens upper and lower extremities.
- Reduces fat from arms, calves and thighs.
- Improve balance.
- Stretches the spine.

Figure 5.8: Garudasana

Indications

- Stiffness of joints of upper and lower extremities.
- Weakness of legs and arms.
- Obesity of arms, thighs and calves.
- Mild giddiness.
- Stiffness of spine.

PARSVOTTANASANA (SIDE STRETCHING POSE)

Technique

- Stand in *Tadasana*.
- Take palms behind the back and join them in prayer position with fingers pointing upwards.
- Take them up as high as possible between the shoulder blades.
- Inhale and keep feet 4 or 4.5 feet apart.
- Exhale and twist to the left by turning left foot out 90 degree and right foot in 70 degree.
- Exhale and bend forward and downward towards the left knee to allow forehead to touch the knee.
- Keep always as high as possible to allow palms to remain together.
- Maintain the pose and breathe normally.
- Inhale and return to original position.
- Repeat pose on the opposite side.

Advantages

- Tones spine.
- Massage abdominal organs.
- Tones neck and larynx.
- Strengthens all the joints.
- Improves blood flow to brain, head, neck and endocrine glands in brain and neck.
- Reduces fat around thighs and abdomen.

Indications

- Stiffness of spine.
- Gastro-intestinal disorder of liver, spleen and spine.

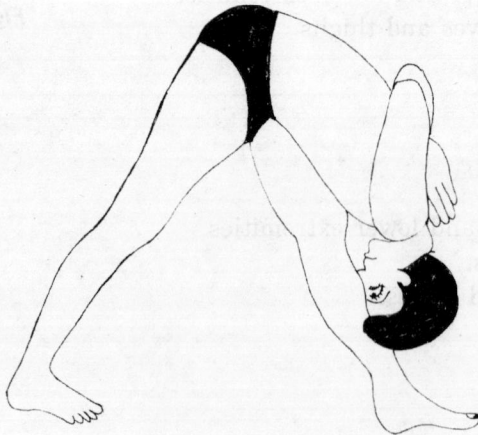

Figure 5.9: Parsvottanasana

- Voice disorders.
- Stiffness of joints.
- Diabetes and thyroid disorders.
- Mental and physical fatigue.
- Obesity of thighs and abdomen.
- Migraine and insomnia.

VIRABHADRASANA–III (VIRABHADRASANA'S POSE III)

Technique

- Stand in *Tadasana*.
- Inhale and keep feet 4 to 4.5 feet apart, raise arms and bring palms together.
- Exhale and twist to the left, turning left foot out 90 degree and right foot on 70 degree.
- Exhale and bend forward left knee to a right angle to be in Virabhadrasana I.
- Exhale and lift right leg and straighten left leg simultaneously, so that the trunk, extended arms and right leg are parallel to the floor.
- Balance body on erect straight left leg, head extended and look forward.
- Maintain the pose and breathe normally.
- Exhale and return to original pose.
- Repeat the pose balancing on the opposite leg.

Advantages

- Strengthens the spine.
- Strengthens legs and reduces obesity around thighs, calves and arms.
- Strengthens neck, abdomen and back muscle.
- Loosen shoulder and hip joints.
- Tones abdominal organs.
- Improves balance, poise and concentration.
- Strengthens inner ears and eyes.

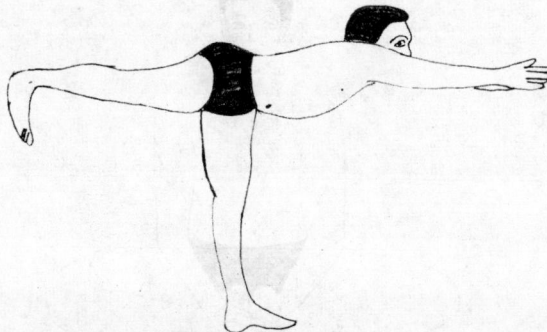

Figure 5.10: Virabhadrasana-III

Indications

- Spondylitis and backaches
- Weak legs.
- Weak abdominal and back muscle.
- Arthritis of joints of upper and lower extremities.
- Gastro-intestinal disorders.
- Mild giddiness.
- Obesity of thighs, calves and arms.
- Weak eyes and ears.

BADDHA KONASANA (COBBLER' S POSE)

Technique

- Sit with back erect and leg straight.
- Exhale, bend knees and bring heels as close as possible to genitals.
- Exhale, allow knees to fall on the sides and bring soles and heels of the feet in contact with each other.
- Catch feet with hands and allow knees and thighs to go down towards floor by pressing thighs down, with elbows and forearms.
- Straighten the back and look straight ahead with eyes relaxed.
- Maintain the pose and breathe normally.
- Exhale and return to the original position.

Advantages

- Relieves pelvic congestion and tones pelvic organs.
- Loosens knee and hip joints.
- Straightens the spine.
- Soothes nerves and the mind.
- Tones gonads.

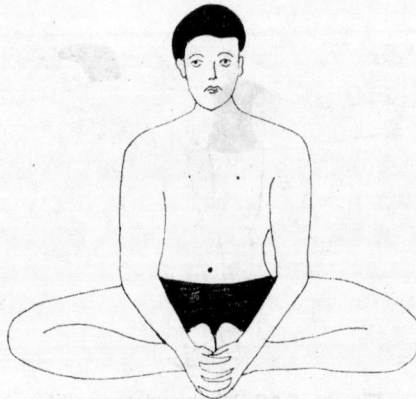

Figure 5.11: Baddha konasana

Indications

- Genito-urinary disorders of prostrate, ovaries, testes and urinary bladder.
- Menstrual irregularities.
- Arthritis of knee and hip joints.
- Sciatica and backache.
- Disorders of sex glands.

VIRASANA (HERO'S POSE)

Technique

- Kneel on the floor with back erect.
- Allow hips to go down and rest them between the feet with toes pointing backwards.
- Keep the back erect and hands resting on the knees, palms facing upwards.
- Join index finger with the thumb to form a ring (Gyana mudra).
- Maintain the pose and breathe normally.
- Bend forward and rest in Adhomukha Virasana pose.

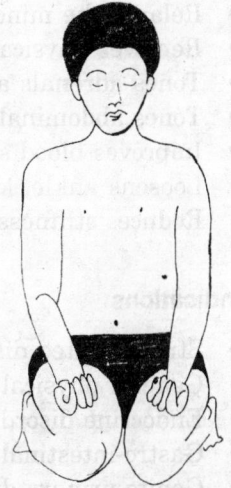

Advantages

- Strengthens the spine.
- Tones stomach and improve digestion.
- Massage pelvic organs.
- Improves flexibility of toes, ankles and the knees.
- Deepens arches of feet.
- Quietness the mind.
- Tones gonads.
- Reduces fat around thighs and calves.

Figure 5.12: Virasana

Indications

- Weak spine.
- Digestive disorders, dyspepsia and indigestion.
- Genito-urinary disorders of prostrate, uterus, testes and ovaries.
- Stiffness of toes, ankles and knees.
- Flat feet.
- Anxiety and tension state.
- Menstrual disorders—Dysmenorrhoea.
- Fat around thighs and calves.

ADHOMUKHA VIRASANA (FACE DOWN HERO'S POSE)

Technique

- Sit in *Virasana*
- Spread the knees a little apart and bend trunk and chest forward between them allowing forehead to rest on the floor.
- Maintain the pose and breathe normally.
- Inhale and return to original pose.

Advantages

- Relaxes the mind.
- Removes physical and mental fatigue.
- Tones adrenals and islets of Langerhans.
- Tones abdominal organs.
- Improves blood supply to brain, head and neck.
- Loosens ankle, knee, hip and shoulder joints.
- Reduces stiffness of spine.

Indications

- Stress related disorders: asthma, diabetes and hypertension.
- General physical or mental fatigue.
- Endocrine disorders of islets of Langerhans, adrenal and gonads.
- Gastro-intestinal disorders of stomach, intestines, liver, spleen and pancreas.
- Genito-urinary disorders of urinary bladder, kidneys, uterus, ovaries and testes.
- Menstrual disorders.
- Stiffness of knee, hips and ankles.
- Stiffness of spine.

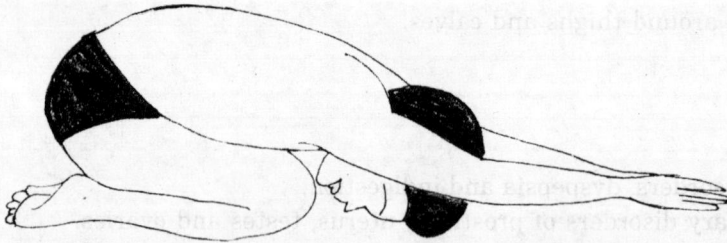

Figure 5.13: Adhomukha Virasana

PADMASANA (LOTUS POSE)

Technique

- Sit with both feet straight.

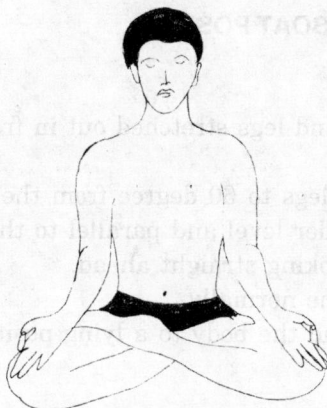

Figure 5.14: Padmasana

- Bend right knee and place outer border of right foot on the left groin.
- Bend left knee and place outer border of left foot on the right groin.
- Try and lift heels further upon the groin and move both knees as close as possible.
- Keep the back straight and shoulder back.
- Rest the hands on the thighs, with the palms facing up, and the index finger and thumb forming a ring (Gyana mudra).
- Maintain the pose and breathe normally.
- Return to original position by retracing the steps.

Advantages

- Tones abdominal organs and spine.
- Tranquilizes mind and heart.
- Opens chest and lungs.
- Increases blood flow to pelvic organs and gonads.
- Loosen knees, ankles and hips.
- Reduces fat around thighs and calves.

Indications

- Mental stress and strain.
- Spondylitis of thoracic and lumbar spine.
- Low backaches.
- Genito-urinary and prostrate disorders.
- Stiffness of knees, ankles and hips.
- Obesity around thighs and calves.

PARIPURNA NAVASANA (FULL BOAT POSE)

Technique

- Sit on floor with back erect and legs stretched out in front, with palms on floor, fingers pointing forward.
- Exhale, lean back and raise legs to 60 degree from the floor.
- Raise arms straight to shoulder level and parallel to the floor.
- Balance on hips with eyes looking straight ahead.
- Maintain the pose and breathe normally.
- Exhale and lower the legs and the body to a lying position and breathe normally.

Advantages

- Reduces load on heart.
- Massages and improves blood flow to abdominal and pelvic organs.
- Increases blood flow to adrenals, islets of Langerhans and gonads.
- Reduces swelling of feet.
- Strengthens thighs and arms.
- Improves balance.

Indications

- Angina and early cardiac problem (done with support to legs and back).
- Gastro-intestinal and pelvic organ disorders, Diarrhoea, dysentery, colitis, dyspepsia, liver, spleen and pancreatic disorders.
- Asthma, diabetes and sexual disorders.
- Oedema of feet due to any cause.
- Weakness of legs and arms.
- Mild giddiness.

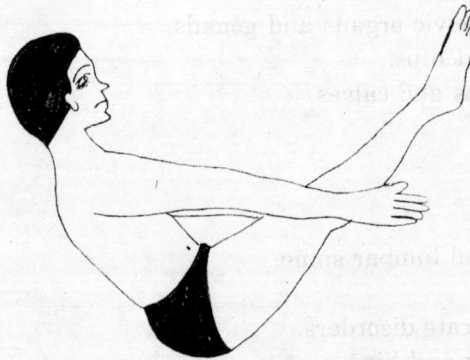

Figure 5.15: Paripurna Navasana

GOMUKHASANA (COW'S FACE POSE)

Technique

- Sit with legs stretched in front and arms on side of hip.
- Raise hip, bend left knee to the left along the floor and place left horizontally under the hips.
- Gently sit over it.
- Bend right knee and place right thigh on top of left thigh with outer border of right foot resting horizontally on the floor, toes pointing backwards.
- Keep back erect.
- Raise left arm, bend it at the elbow and place palm facing forward between two shoulder blades.
- Take right arm behind; bend it at the elbow and place palm facing backward between the shoulder blades.
- Grip fingers of both hands and bring hands closer to each other by allowing both elbows more backward.
- Maintain the pose and breathe normally.
- Exhale and return to original pose.

Advantages

- Loosen all small and big joints.
- Expand chest and lungs.
- Massages and improves blood flow to pelvic organs.
- Reduce obesity around thigh, leg and arm.
- Stretches spine.
- Tones gonads.
- Strengthens shoulders, arms and thighs.

Indications

- Arthritis.
- Respiratory disorders, asthma, bronchitis.
- Genito-urinary disorders of urinary bladder, uterus, and prostate.
- Obesity around thighs, calves, and arms.
- Stiffness of spine.
- Disorders of sex glands.
- Weak shoulders, arms and thigh.

Figure 5.16: Gomukhasana

SIMHASANA-II (LION POSE)

Technique

- Sit in *Padmasana*.
- Place extended arms on side of thigh and raise trunk up on knees shifting the arms to the front and placing palms on the floor.

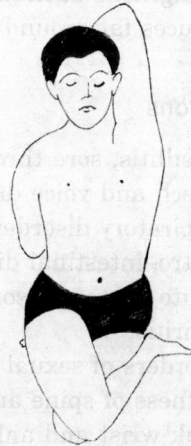

- Push pubis forward towards the floor by shifting the palms further forward on the floor to stretch the back and make it concave.
- Open the mouth and stretch the tongue out towards the chin as much as possible.
- Look towards the tip of the nose and breathe through the mouth.
- Maintain the pose and breathe.
- Exhale and return to original pose.

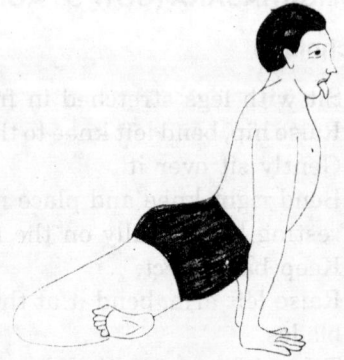

Figure 5.17: Simhasana-II

Advantages

- Tones and clears the tongue, throat and larynx.
- Removes bad breathe.
- Improves speech.
- Expands chest and lungs.
- Tones abdominal and pelvic organs.
- Strengthens all joints.
- Tones adrenals, islets of Langerhans and gonads.
- Strengthens back muscles and spine.
- Reduces fat around the hips, thighs and arms.

Indications

- Tonsillitis, sore throats, laryngitis.
- Speech and voice disorders.
- Respiratory disorders, asthma, and bronchitis
- Gastro–intestinal disorders of liver, stomach, and intestine.
- Genito-urinary disorders of urinary bladder, uterus, and prostate.
- Arthritis,
- Disorders of sexual glands and diabetes.
- Stiffness of spine and backache.
- Weak wrist and ankle.
- Obesity around thighs, arms, and hips.

PARIGHASANA (GATE POSE)

Technique

- Kneel on knees with thighs and trunk erect.
- Stretches left leg to left in line with the trunk, knee pointing upwards, and raise both arms up parallel to the floor.
- Exhale, bend trunk and left arm to the left in line with the left leg, and rest the forearm on the shin with palm facing upwards.

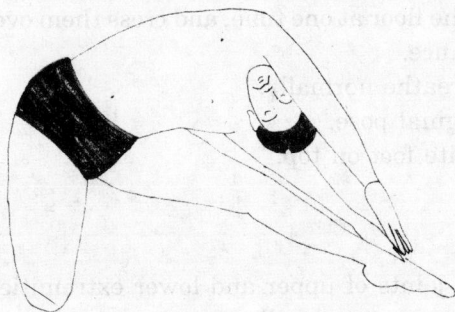

Figure 5.18: Parighasana

- Take right arm over the head with palm facing downwards and touch left palm without bending forward.
- Maintain the pose and breathe normally.
- Repeat pose on the opposite side.

Advantages

- Tones up paravertebral muscles and spine.
- Massages abdominal and pelvic organs.
- Strengthens all muscles and joints of upper and lower extremities
- Tones adrenals, islets of Langerhans and gonads.
- Extends and expands sides of chest and lungs.
- Reduces fat around the waist, thighs and calves.

Indications

- Low and mid backaches
- Gastro-intestinal disorders of stomach, liver, spleen and intestine.
- Genito-urinary disorders of kidneys, urinary bladder, uterus and prostate.
- Arthritis.
- Diabetes, asthma, and sexual disorders.
- Obesity around the waist, thighs and calves.
- Weakness of legs.

BHUJAPIDASANA (KNEE SHOULDER POSE)

Technique

- Stand in *Tadasana* with feet one foot apart.
- Bend trunk forward, bend knees and place hands on floor between legs as far back as possible.
- Bring palms forward on outer sides of feet, and rest thighs on upper arm as high as possible.

- Exhale and raise feet off the floor at one time, and cross them over each other at the ankles.
- Straighten arms and balance.
- Maintain the pose and breathe normally.
- Exhale and return to original pose.
- Repeat asana with opposite foot on top.

Advantages

- Strengthens muscles and joints of upper and lower extremities.
- Improves balance, concentration and will power.
- Strengthens inner ears and eyes.
- Tones and strengthens abdominal organs and muscles.
- Tones adrenal glands.
- Reduces obesity around arms and thighs.

Indications:

- Weakness of upper and lower extremities.
- Stiffness of extremity joints.
- Lack of concentration and diffidence.
- Weak abdominal muscles.
- Gastro-intestinal disorders of stomach, intestines, liver and spleen.
- Diabetes.
- Obesity around arms and thighs.

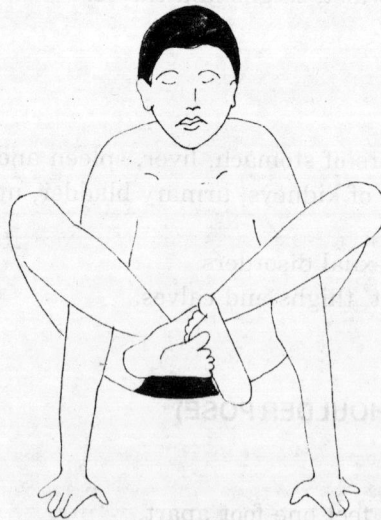

Figure 5.19: Bhujapidasana

BAKASANA (CRANE POSE)

Technique

- Stand in *Tadasana*.
- Bend the knees and squat.
- Widen knees, bend trunk forwards and allow shins to contact the upper arm.
- Widen elbows and place palms on the floor, fingers pointing forward.
- Bend trunk and chest further forward between the arms, raise the hips and heels up, and rest the shins on the arms as high and close to the armpit as possible.
- Exhale and lift feet up, at one time, straighten the arms and balance on hands.
- Maintain the pose and breathe normally.
- Exhale and return to original position.

Advantages

- Improves balance and concentration.
- Strengthens muscles and joints of upper extremities including palms and fingers.
- Tones abdominal muscle.
- Strengthens inner ears and eyes.

Indications

- Stiffness of extremity joints.
- Weak upper extremities
- Poor concentration and diffidence.
- Flabby and weak abdomen.

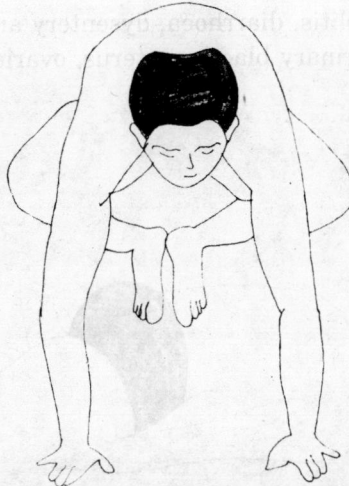

Figure 5.20: Bakasana

SUPTA BADDHA KONASANA (COBBLER'S POSE IN LYING POSITION)

Technique

- Sit in *Baddha Konasana*.
- Recline back and allow head and back to come in contact with floor.
- Push hands under the thighs, hold ankles and pull them up so that the heels touch the anal region.
- Keep outer sides of knees in full contact with the floor.
- Keep arms on side of thighs with palms facing the ceiling.
- Maintain the pose and breathe normally.
- Exhale and return to original pose.

Advantages

- Tranquillizes mind.
- Expands chest and lungs.
- Tones abdominal organs.
- Relieves pelvic congestion.
- Relieves congestion in gonads.
- Lowers blood pressure.
- Loosens knee and hip joints.

Indications

- General physical or mental fatigue.
- Insomnia, anxiety and tension states.
- Respiratory disorders, asthma and bronchitis.
- Gastro-intestinal disorders, colitis, diarrhoea, dysentery and peptic ulcer.
- Genito-urinary disorders of urinary bladder, uterus, ovaries, testes and prostate.
- Menstrual disorders.
- Disorders of sex glands.
- High blood pressure.
- Stiff knee and hip joints.

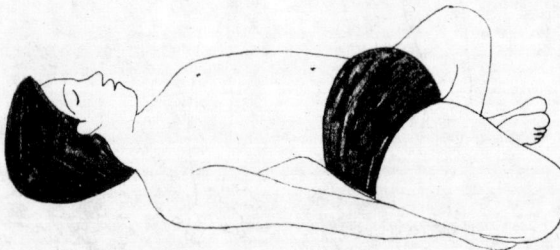

Figure 5.21: Supta Baddha Konasana

SUPTA VIRASANA (HERO'S POSE IN LYING POSITION)

Technique

- Sit in *Virasana*.
- Recline back and rest elbows on the floor.
- Extend the arms at one time and allow the head and back to rest on the floor.
- Take arms over the head and straighten them.
- Maintain the pose and breathe normally.
- Exhale and return to original pose, lean forwards and rest in *Adhomukha Virasana* pose.

Advantages

- Expands chest and lungs.
- Tones heart and abdominal organs.
- Reduces congestion in pelvic organs.
- Straightens and tones the spine.
- Relax mind.
- Loosen ankle, knee, hip and shoulder.
- Tones adrenals, islets of Langerhans and gonads.
- Reduces fat around thighs and calves.

Indications

- Respiratory disorders—asthma, bronchitis, and chronic obstructive lung disease.
- Gastro-intestinal disorders—dyspepsia, diarrhoea and colitis.
- Menstrual disorders.
- Postural defects of spine.
- Anxiety and mental tension.
- Stiffness of ankle, knee, hip and shoulder.
- Endocrine disorder—diabetes, asthma, and disorders of sexual gland.
- Obesity of thighs and calves.
- Preparatory posture for Pranayama.

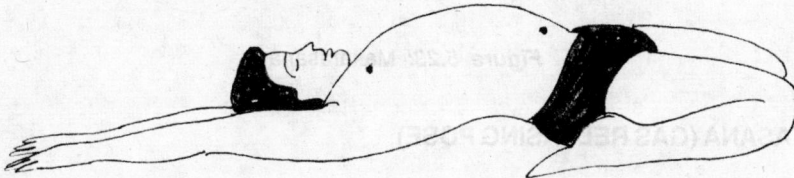

Figure 5.22: Supta Virasana

MAKARASANA (CROCODILE POSE)

Technique

- Lie on belly with chin on floor and crossed forearms above the head.
- Inhale, raise chest, and bring arms in line with shoulders and place forehead on the crossed forearms.
- Keep legs astride as far as possible, with inner borders of feet touching the floor.
- Keep chest above ground and abdomen in full contact with the floor.
- Do abdominal breathing, with abdomen moving towards the floor during inhalation and away from the floor during exhalation.
- Exhale and return to original pose.

Advantages

- Reduces stress and fatigue.
- Strengthens the diaphragm.
- Improves diaphragmatic breathing.
- Massage chest and abdominal organs, heart, lungs, stomach, liver, spleen intestine, and gall bladder.
- Tones the heart.
- Loosens shoulder, hip and ankle joint.

Indications

- Stress related disorders—hypertension, peptic ulcer, colitis, diabetes and asthma.
- General physical and mental fatigue.
- Gastro-intestinal disorders, dyspepsia, peptic ulcer and constipation.
- Respiratory disorders—chronic bronchitis and asthma.
- Stiffness of shoulder, hip and ankle.

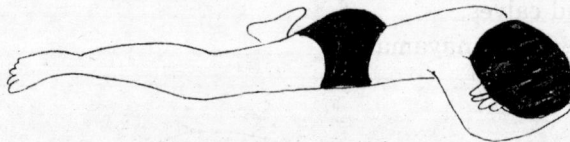

Figure 5.23: Makarasana

PAWANMUKTASANA (GAS RELEASING POSE)

Technique

- Lie on back with feet together.
- Exhale and bend both knees and hold shins down with locked hands or crossed forearms.
- Exhale and press thigh gently towards lower abdomen.

- Exhale and raise head up and touch forehead to knees.
- Maintain the pose and breathe normally.
- Inhale and return to original pose.

Note—If you have a sore back, use one pillow under the hips and another between the neck and shoulder blades to relieve strain on back.

Advantages

- Massages abdominal organs—stomach and intestine.
- Massages endocrine glands—thyroid, adrenals parathyroid, islets of Langerhans and gonads.
- Tones the spine.
- Loosen knee, hip, elbow and finger joints.
- Reduces obesity of abdomen, thighs and arms.
- Strengthens abdominal and neck muscles.

Indications

- Digestive disorders—dyspepsia, flatulence, constipation and colitis.
- Gallbladder, spleen and liver disorders.
- Thyroid, parathyroid and gonad disorders.
- Diabetes
- Weak spine
- Arthritis
- Obesity around abdomen, thighs and arms
- Weak abdominal and neck muscles.

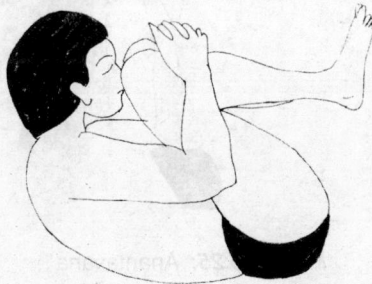

Figure 5.24: Pawanmuktasana

ANANTASANA (GOD VISHNU'S RESTING POSE)

Technique

- Lie on back with feet together.
- Turn body to left and lie on left side with body in full contact with the floor.
- Extend left arm upwards, bend elbow, and rest portion of the head behind the left ear on the palm.

- Bend right knee and hold big toe with the fingers on the right hand.
- Exhale and extend right leg and arm vertically upward simultaneously till knee and the elbow are locked.
- Maintain the pose and breathe normally.
- Exhale and return to original pose.
- Repeat pose on opposite side.

Advantages

- Strengthens joints of upper and lower extremities
- Soothes mind and nerves.
- Stretches and relaxes nerves of legs and arms
- Improves venous drainage from legs and arms.
- Tones the lungs and abdominal organs.

Indications

- Arthritis and sciatica.
- Mental stress and strain.
- Stress related disorders—hypertension, peptic ulcer and colitis.
- General physical and mental fatigue.
- Genito-urinary disorders of uterus, urinary bladder, testes, ovaries and prostate.
- Disorders of sex glands.
- Oedema of legs or arms.
- Menstrual disorders.

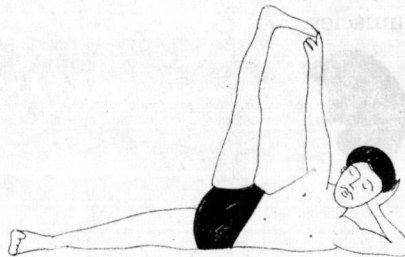

Figure 5.25: Anantasana

SALAMBA SARVANGASANA (SHOULDER STAND POSE)

Technique

- Lie on the back with feet together and palms close to the body facing the floor.
- Bend the knees and rest thighs on the lower abdomen.
- Exhale and lift hips and thighs to 60° and support them with the palms and fingers by bending arms at the elbows.
- Exhale and lift trunk and thighs to a vertical position supporting the back with palms.
- Slide palms down on the back towards the head till chest touches chin.

- Straighten the legs and point toes upward.
- Maintain the pose and breathe normally.
- Exhale and slide down to original pose.

Advantages

- Improves blood to pituitary, pineal, thyroid and parathyroid gland.
- Improves blood flow to head, neck and brain.
- Improves blood flow to all the sense organs—eyes, nose, ears, tongue, and the skin of the face.
- Reduces swelling of feet and legs and pelvic congestion.
- Replaces sagging abdominal organs back to their position.
- Strengthens joints of upper extremities.
- Reduces mental and physical fatigue.

Indications

- Pituitary, thyroid, parathyroid and gonad disorders.
- Insomnia, poor memory and concentration.
- Oedema of feet and legs and piles.
- Mild giddiness.
- Gastro-intestinal disorders of stomach and intestines.
- Genito-urinary disorders of urinary bladder, uterus and prostate.
- Physical and mental fatigue.
- Weak joints of upper extremities.
- Preparatory posture of Sirsasana.

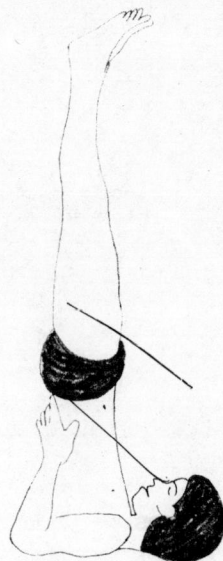

Figure 5.26: Salamba Sarvangasana

ADHOMUKHA SVANASANA (DOG, FACE DOWN POSE)

Technique

- Lie on your belly with forehead on the floor, feet one-foot apart, and hands close to your shoulder with the elbow bent vertically.
- Raise the hips up; still higher by straightening the knees allowing the tailbone to become the highest point.
- Move shoulders and chest downwards and backwards towards thighs.
- Stretch the legs by allowing the heels to move downward maintaining the tailbone at the same height.
- Allow the head to relax and to rest on the floor or on one or two folded blankets as required.
- Maintain the pose and breathe normally.
- Exhale and return to original pose.

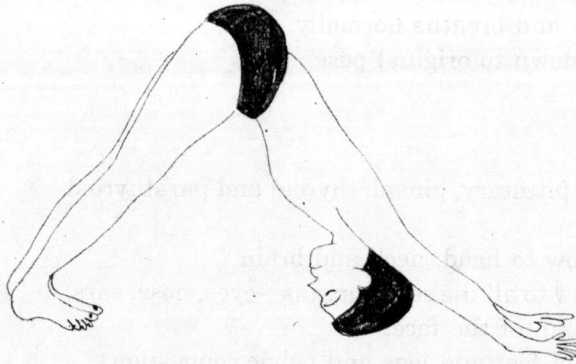

Figure 5.27: Adhomukha Svanasana

Advantages

- Improves blood flow to brain, head, neck, fingers and toes.
- Improves blood flow to pituitary, pineal, thyroid and parathyroid glands and reduces congestion in gonads.
- Reduces congestion in pelvic and abdominal organ.
- Drains the lungs.
- Strengthens muscles and joints of upper and lower extremities.
- Reduces fat in upper and lower extremities.
- Increases stamina.
- Improves memory, concentration, intellect and creativity.

Indications

- Hair loss and insomnia
- Thyroid, parathyroid and sexual disorders.
- Respiratory disorders, chronic bronchitis.
- Genito-urinary and menstrual disorders.
- Arthritis.
- Weakness or obesity of arms and legs.
- Stress related disorders.
- Poor memory and concentration.

PRASARITA PADOTTANASANA (WIDE LEGS STRETCHING POSE)
Technique

- Stand in *Tadasana*
- Spread legs 4 feet apart and place hands on waist.

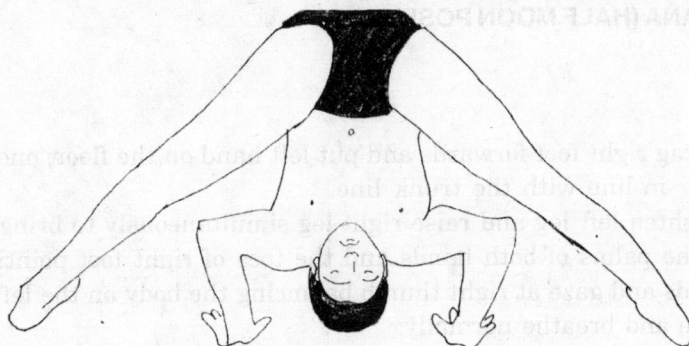

Figure 5.28: Prasarita Padottanasana

- Exhale, bend forwards with neck extended and back concave, and place palms on floor between the feet.
- Exhale and bend elbows to allow head to rest on the floor between the two palms.
- Keep medial arches of feet raised.
- Maintain the pose and breathe normally.
- Inhale and return to original pose.

Advantages

- Improves blood flow to head, neck and trunk.
- Improves blood flow to pituitary, pineal, thyroid, parathyroid and thymus glands.
- Reduces mental and physical fatigue.
- Strengthens legs and reduces fat around thighs.
- Strengthens ankle and wrist joints.
- Reduces congestion in abdominal and pelvic organs and gonads.
- Drains out secretions from lungs.

Indications

- Migraine, insomnia, lack of concentration, poor memory and mental fatigue.
- Pituitary, thyroid and parathyroid disorders.
- Physical or mental fatigue.
- Weakness of legs and fat around the thighs.
- Weakness of ankle, wrist and elbow joints.
- Menstrual disorders.
- Disorders of sex glands.
- Pelvic organ disorders of urinary bladder, uterus and prostate.

ARDHACHANDRASANA (HALF MOON POSE)

Technique

- Do *Trikonasana*
- Bend left knee, drag right foot forwards and put left hand on the floor, one-foot away and slightly outside or in line with the trunk line.
- Exhale and straighten left leg and raise right leg simultaneously to bring it in line with the trunk, with the palms of both hands and the toes of right foot pointing forwards.
- Turn head upwards and gaze at right thumb balancing the body on the left hand and leg.
- Maintain the pose and breathe normally.
- Exhale and return to the original pose.
- Repeat the pose on the opposite side.

Advantages

- Reduces congestion in abdominal and pelvic organs.
- Drains phlegm (thick mucous) from lungs.
- Improves balance and poise.
- Strengthens inner ears and eyes.
- Improves blood circulation to the head, neck, hypothalamus and endocrine glands in brain and neck.
- Helps venous drainage from extremities.
- Tones spine.
- Strengthens legs, knees and hip joints.
- Reduces fat around thighs.

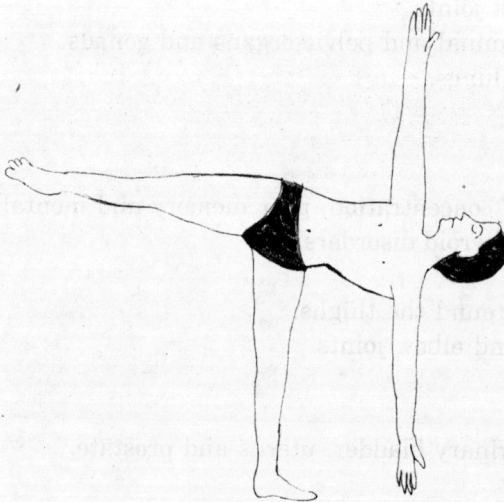

Figure 5.29: Ardhachandrasana

Indications

- Genito-urinary disorders of urinary bladder and uterus.
- Gastro-intestinal disorders, indigestion and dyspepsia.
- Chronic bronchitis
- Mild giddiness
- Poor memory, concentration, and eyesight.
- Insomnia and falling hair.
- Endocrine disorders of pituitary, thyroid, and parathyroid glands.
- Arthritis.
- Stiffness of spine.
- Obesity of thighs and weakness of legs.

SETU BANDHA SARVANGASANA (BRIDGE POSE)

Technique

- Do *Sarvangasana*
- Bend the knees and allow trunk to fall to the floor over the wrists, firmly supporting the lower dorsal spine with the palms.
- Straightens the legs slowly at one time and keep feet together.
- Maintain the pose and breathe normally.
- Exhale and gradually lower the body to a lying position and breathe normally.

Note—If you can't do this independently use a long bench to support the hips and legs.

Advantages

- Tones lumbo-dorsal spine.
- Broadens chest and expands lungs.
- Massages abdominal and pelvic organ.
- Improves blood flow to neck, brain, and hypothalamus.
- Soothes nervous system and mind.
- Increases blood supply and massages thyroid and parathyroid gland.
- Reduces fat around things and arms.
- Strengthens arms, wrists and ankles.
- Reduces congestion of gonads.

Indications

- Spondylitis and backaches.
- Respiratory disorders, asthma and bronchitis.
- Gastro-intestinal and pelvic organ disorders.
- General apathy and mental depression.
- Insomnia, poor memory, lack of concentration.

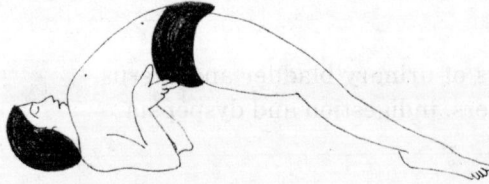

Figure 5.30: Setu Bandha Sarvangasana

- Thyroid and parathyroid dysfunction.
- Disorders of sex glands.
- Weakness of arms, wrists and ankles.
- Fat around thighs and arms.

HALASANA (PLOUGH POSE)

Technique

- Do *Salamba Sarvangasana*
- Release chin lock and lower trunk and legs gently to the floor on the head side, bringing arms upward under the legs at the same time.
  Note—If this is not possible, do half Halasana with the legs resting on a bench or a stool of the appropriate height.
- Raise trunk further up to vertical level by contracting muscles of the thighs, and by placing hands in middle of back and lifting it.
- Release hands and stretch them back in a direction opposite to that of the legs.
- Maintain the pose and breathe normally.
- Exhale and return to *Sarvangasana* and then slowly lower the trunk and legs to the floor.

Advantages

- Reduces stiffness of shoulders and back.
- Massages abdominal organs.
- Relieves congestion from pelvic organs and gonads.
- Tones endocrine glands, pituitary, pineal, thyroid, parathyroid, adrenals and islets of Langerhans.

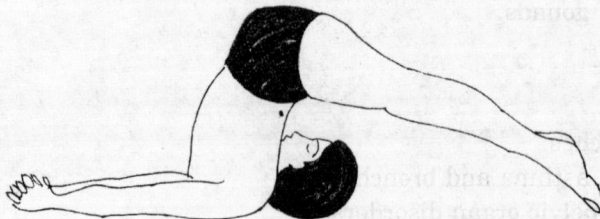

Figure 5.31: Halasana

- Relaxes and rejuvenates the mind.
- Loosens joints of upper and lower limbs.
- Improves circulation of brain, hypothalamus, head and neck.

Indications

- Stiffness of back and shoulders.
- Gastro-intestinal disorders of liver, spleen and pancreas.
- Genito-urinary disorders of urinary bladder, prostate, ovaries and testes.
- Stress related diseases--diabetes, asthma and colitis.
- Pituitary, thyroid and parathyroid disorders.
- Diabetes.
- Mental tension, anxiety and depression.

SALAMBA SIRSASANA (HEAD STAND POSE)

Technique

- Kneel behind a folded blanket, bend forward, place arms on blanket parallel to each other and in line with the shoulders.
- Without shifting elbows, bring hands close to each other and interlock fingers to form a cup, resting on the inner borders of the palms.
- Place crown of head on blanket so that back of head fits snugly in the cup of the palms.
- Raise knees and hips up and walk in towards trunk, allowing it to become as vertical as possible.
- Exhale and with a gentle swing, lift feet off the floor with bent knees.
- Straighten thighs first, followed by the legs, and balance body on crown of head keeping legs, trunk, neck and head in one line.
- Maintain the pose and breathe normally.
- Exhale and return to original position.

Advantages

- Improves blood flow to pituitary, pineal, thyroid and parathyroid glands.
- Removes congestion from gonads.
- Improves blood flow to brain, head, neck and hypothalamus.
- Improves balance, concentration, confidence, will-power and creativity.
- Strengthens inner ears and eyes.
- Helps venous drainage from lower extremities and pelvis.
- Replaces sagging abdominal organs to their original place

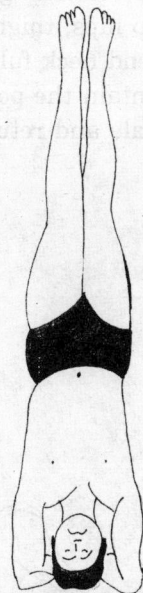

Figure 5.32: Salamba Sirsasana

- Drains secretions from lungs and improves ventilation.
- Improves alignment of back and spine.

Indications

- Endocrine disorders and poor body immunity.
- Weak eyes, inner ears and other senses.
- Poor memory, intelligence, concentration and will-power.
- Baldness, insomnia and migraine.
- Varicose veins, oedema of feet and piles.
- Inguinal hernia, constipation.
- Poor lung power, chronic coughs, colds, tonsillitis
- Physical and mental fatigue.
- Stiffness of back and spine.

BHUJANGASANA (COBRA POSE)

Technique

- Lie on belly with forehead on floor and arms close to the chest.
- Bend elbows and bring hands close to the shoulders, with fingers spread out.
- Inhale and raise head, neck, chest and upper belly off the floor, keeping lower belly and pubis on the floor.
- Keep remaining portion of the body in close contact with the floor.
- Keep hips, thighs and knees firm and contracted.
- Extend neck fully, look towards the sky and brace shoulders backwards.
- Maintain the pose and breathe normally.
- Exhale and return to original pose.

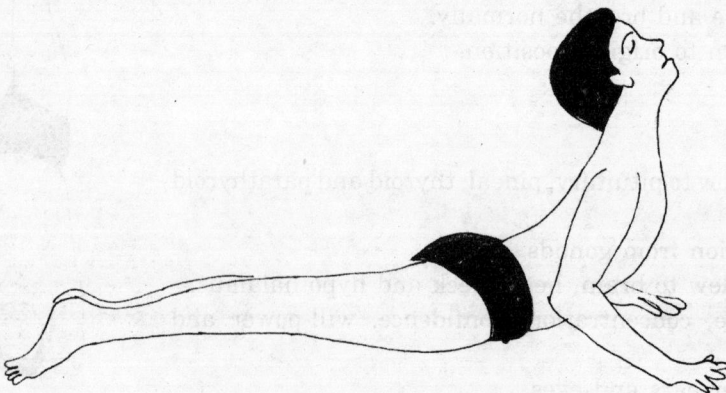

Figure 5.33: Bhujangasana

Advantages

- Strengthens complete spine, posterior spinal muscles and ligaments.
- Tones larynx, heart and neck muscle.
- Broadens chest.
- Stimulates abdominal and pelvic organs.
- Stimulates thyroid, parathyroid, adrenal glands and islets of Langerhans.
- Strengthens joints of upper extremities.
- Tones hips and thighs muscles.

Indications

- Cervical and thoracic spondylitis
- Upper and mid backache
- Early slipped discs and sciatica.
- Voice disorders.
- Asthma and bronchitis.
- Abdominal and pelvic organ disorders.
- Thyroid and parathyroid disorders, asthma and diabetes.
- Arthritis of upper extremity joints.

SALABHASANA (LOCUST POSE)

Technique

- Lie on belly with forehead on the floor, feet together with toes pointing backwards and arms close to body, palm facing upwards.
- Inhale and raise head, chest and thighs up simultaneously, as high as possible along with the arms pointing towards the toes at shoulder level without bending knees.
- Body should be resting only on the abdomen.
- Contract hip muscles and close the anus.
- Keep elbows and knees locked.
- Maintain the pose and breathe normally.
- Exhale and return to original pose.
- Keep face sideways on the floor, arms on side of thighs and breathe normally.

Advantages

- Tones complete spine.
- Tones abdominal organs and heart.
- Expands chest and lungs.
- Tones thyroid, parathyroid, adrenals, islets of Langerhans and gonads.
- Strengthens muscles of back, thighs, arms, neck, and front of abdomen.
- Strengthens all joints of upper and lower extremities.

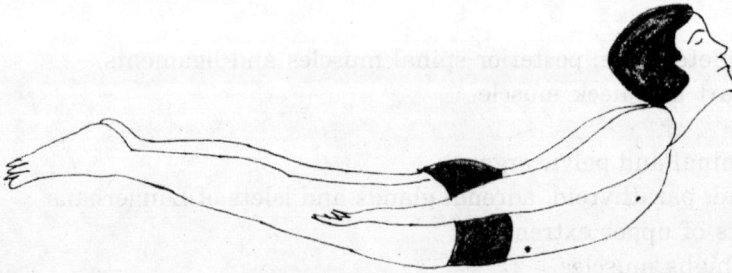

Figure 5.34: Salabhasana

Indications

- Cervical thoracic and lumbar spondylitis.
- Upper, mid and low backaches.
- Gastro-intestinal disorders of liver, spleen, gall bladder and stomach.
- Asthma, bronchitis and emphysema.
- Thyroid and parathyroid disorders.
- Diabetes and disorders of sex glands.
- Protruding and weak abdomen.
- Arthritis.

URDHVA MUKHA SVANASANA (DOG FACE UPWARD POSE)

Technique

- Lie on the belly with forehead on the floor, feet one foot apart and hands close to the waist, with elbow bent.
- Raise and extend head, neck, chest, abdomen, thighs, knees and legs completely by gradually straightening the arms.
- Maintain the pose by resting only on the palms and extended toes.
- Push chest forwards and tighten the hip muscle.
- Maintain the pose and breathe normally
- Exhale and return to original pose.
- Keep face sideways on the floor, arms on the side of the thighs, palms facing upwards and breathe normally.

Advantages

- Tones complete spine and heart.
- Expand chest and lungs.
- Tones thyroid, adrenals, islets of Langerhans and gonads.
- Strengthens all the joints and muscles of upper and lower extremities.
- Reduces fat around the abdomen, arms and legs.

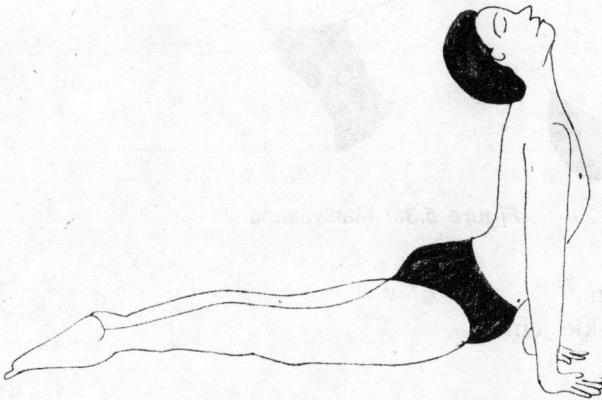

Figure 5.35: Urdhva Mukha Svanasana

Indications

- Spondylitis
- Respiratory diseases—asthma, emphysema, chronic bronchitis.
- Gastro-intestinal disorders of liver, spleen, stomach and intestine.
- Genito-urinary disorders of urinary bladder, uterus and prostate.
- Thyroid, adrenal and gonad disorders.
- Diabetes.
- Arthritis.
- Obesity around abdomen, arms or legs.

MATSYASANA (FISH POSE)

Technique

- Sit in *Padmasana*
- Exhale and arch the back to lower the head, neck and back, till crown of the head rests on the floor.
- Hold the feet in your hands and increases the arch of the back and the chest.
- Bend the arms, hold elbows and rest the arms behind the head.
- Maintain the pose and breathe normally.
- Exhale and return to original pose.

Advantages

- Tones cervical and thoracic spine.
- Expands chest and lungs.
- Massages thyroid and parathyroid.
- Tones larynx and heart.

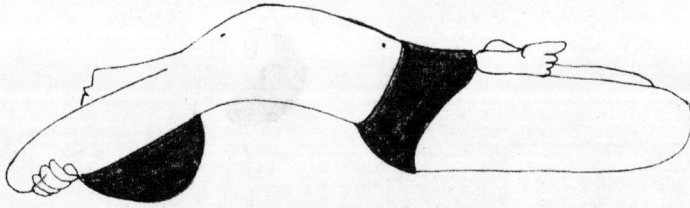

Figure 5.36: Matsyasana

- Relieves pelvic congestion.
- Loosens shoulder and ankle joints.

Indications

- Cervical and thoracic spondylitis.
- Respiratory disorders: asthma, bronchitis.
- Thyroid and parathyroid disorders.
- Voice disorders.
- Menstrual disorders.
- Stiffness of shoulder and ankle joints.
- Counter pose to *Sarvangasana.*

USTRASANA (CAMEL POSE)

Technique

- Kneel with thighs and trunk erect, and hands on hips.
- Exhale and arch backwards.
- Arch more by sliding hands down on back of thighs, extending the head and neck backwards.
- Exhale and release hands one at a time to hold the heels.
- Press heels with hands to push spine towards thighs which are kept erect.
- Maintain the pose and breathe normally.
- Return to original pose by replacing hands on thighs and walk up with the hands to allow head, neck, trunk and spine to come in one line.
- Bend knees and sit in *Virasana.*
- Bend forward to rest forehead on the floor in *Adhomukha Virasana.*

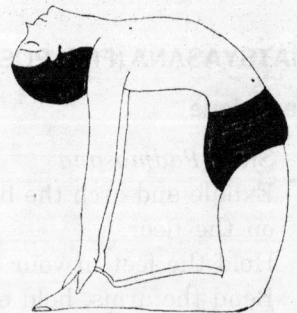

Figure 5.37: Ustrasana

Advantages

- Tones complete spine.
- Broadens chest and expands lungs.

- Tones larynx, heart and neck muscles.
- Tones abdominal and pelvic organs.
- Stimulates all endocrine glands.
- Strengthens shoulder and hip joints.
- Reduces fat around thigh.

Indications

- Spondylitis of cervical, thoracic and lumbar spine.
- Respiratory disorders—asthma, bronchitis, and emphysema.
- Voice disorders.
- Gastro-intestinal disorders—dyspepsia, constipation, colitis, liver and gall bladder disorders.
- Genito-urinary disorders of kidney, urinary bladder, ovaries, testes and prostate.
- Thyroid and parathyroid disorders.
- Diabetes.
- Stiffness of shoulder and hip.
- Obesity around thigh.

DHANURASANA (BOW POSE)

Technique

- Lie down on belly with forehead on the floor, arms on side of thighs and feet slightly apart.
- Bend knees and hold ankles with outstretched hands.
- Exhale completely and lift knees and chest up simultaneously by pulling on the shins with the arms.
- Raise thighs and chest further upward by allowing the feet to move towards the ceiling and allowing the head to be extended back as far as possible.
- Approximate ankles, knees and thighs.
- Maintain the pose and breathe normally.
- Exhale and return to original pose.

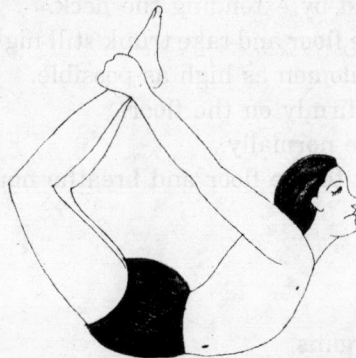

Figure 5.38: Dhanurasana

Advantages

- Brings elasticity and flexibility to spine.
- Massages abdominal and pelvic organs.
- Expands chest and lungs.
- Tones heart, adrenals, gonads, islets of Langerhans.
- Strengthens upper and lower extremities.
- Loosens joints of extremities.
- Reduces fat around the waist, thighs and arms.
- Strengthens neck.

Indications

- Backache.
- Cervical, thoracic and lumbar spondylitis.
- Gastro-intestinal disorders of liver, spleen and intestine.
- Respiratory disorders—chronic bronchitis, and asthma
- Genito-urinary disorders of kidneys, urinary bladder, uterus sex glands and prostate.
- Diabetes, asthma and sexual disorders.
- Weakness of upper and lower extremities.
- Obesity around waist, thighs and arms.

URDHVA DHANURASANA (UPWARD BOW POSE)

Technique

- Lie on back with feet 6 inches apart.
- Bend knees and bring feet close to the thighs.
- Take arms over the head and place them close to the shoulders with elbows bent and fingers pointing towards feet.
- Exhale and raise trunk and chest, by putting pressure of hands and feet on the ground and opening up elbows and knees partially.
- Place crown of head on ground by extending the neck.
- Exhale and raise head from the floor and take trunk still higher by straightening the arms and raising the thighs and abdomen as high as possible.
- Keep palms and soles of feet firmly on the floor.
- Maintain the pose and breathe normally.
- Exhale, lower the body gently to the floor and breathe normally.

Advantages

- Strengthens complete spine.
- Tones heart and abdominal organs.
- Strengthens all joints.

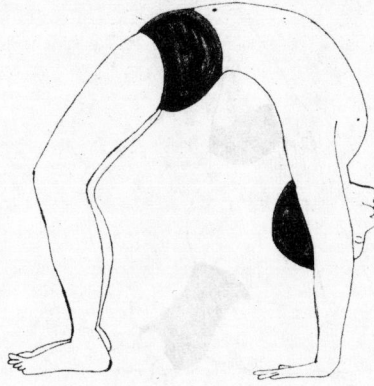

Figure 5.39: Urdhva Dhanurasana

- Stretches and strengthens muscles of frontal abdomen, extremities and the back.
- Expands chest and lungs.
- Reduces fat around abdomen and extremities.

Indications.

- Spondylitis, backaches, early disc problems and sciatica.
- Gastro-intestinal disorders of liver, pancreas, spleen, stomach and gall bladder.
- Weakness of muscles and joints of upper and lower extremities.
- Respiratory disorders—asthma and bronchitis.
- Endocrinological disorders—diabetes, thyroid and disorders of the sex glands.
- Genito-urinary disorders and prostate.
- Obesity.

EKA-PADA RAJAKAPOTASANA-I (PIGEON POSE)

Technique

- Sit with legs straight.
- Bend left knee parallel to the floor and touch heel to right groin.
- Take right leg back and stretch it straight with toes pointing backwards.
- Put hands on waist and throw the head back.
- Place hands on floor, bend the right knee and bring foot close to the head.
- Exhale and take both arms at one time over the head, to hold the right foot.
- Maintain the pose and breathe normally.
- Exhale and return to original pose.
- Repeat the pose on opposite side.

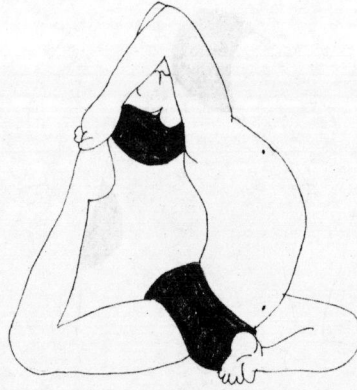

Figure 5.40: Eka Pada Rajakapotasan-I

Advantages

- Rejuvenates lower spine.
- Broadens chest and expands lungs.
- Strengthens larynx.
- Tone all endocrine glands, abdominal and pelvic organs.
- Strengthens neck, shoulder, groin and thighs.

Indications

- Spondylitis and lumbo-sacral backache.
- Gastro-intestinal and pelvic organ disorders.
- Asthma and bronchitis.
- Voice disorders.
- Thyroid and parathyroid disorders.
- Diabetes and disorders of sex glands.
- Arthritis.
- Weak neck, shoulders and thighs.
- Obesity of abdomen and thighs.

BHARAD VAJARASANA-I (BHARAD VAJ'S POSE)

Technique

- Sit with feet straight and spine erect.
- Bend both knees so that they point to the right and the feet to the left and raise the left arm up.
- Exhale and twist trunk towards the right, bring down and push left hand under right thigh, with palm facing the floor.
- Take right hand behind back, and hold left arm.

- Look over the left shoulder.
- Maintain the pose and breathe normally.
- Inhale and return to original pose.
- Repeat pose on the opposite side.

Advantages

- Tones complete spine.
- Massages abdominal organs, especially kidney.
- Opens chest and lungs.
- Loosens all joints.
- Massages endocrine glands, adrenals, islets of Langerhans and gonads.
- Narrows the waist.
- Tones neck muscles, larynx and heart.

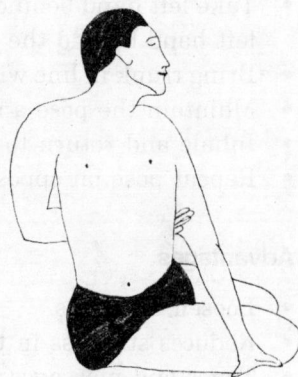

Figure 5.41: Bharad Vajarasana-I

Indications

- Lumbago and spondylitis.
- Genito-urinary disorders of ovaries, testes, prostate, urinary bladder and kidney.
- Gastro-intestinal disorders of liver, spleen, intestine and pancreas.
- Respiratory disorders—chronic bronchitis, asthma and bronchiectasis.
- Arthritis.
- Diabetes.
- Obesity.
- Voice disorders.

MARICYASANA-I (SAGE MARICH'S POSE)

Technique

- Sit with legs straight and spine erect.
- Bend right knee vertically and place right heel close to right thigh.
- Take right arm over the right knee to hold the left toes and twist towards the left.

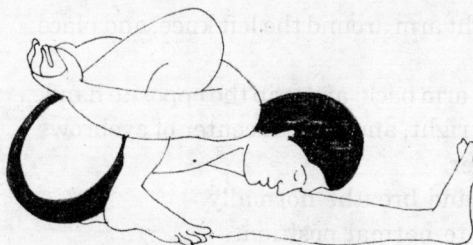

Figure 5.42: Maricyasana-I

- Take left hand behind the back, and revolve the right hand around the right shin, to hold left hand behind the back.
- Bring trunk in line with the left thigh and bend forwards to touch chin to left thigh or shin.
- Maintain the pose and breathe normally.
- Inhale and return to original position.
- Repeat pose on opposite side.

Advantages

- Loosen all joints.
- Reduces stiffness in the spine.
- Tones and massages abdominal organs and endocrine gland.
- Reduces fat around thighs and abdomen.
- Reduces physical and mental stress.

Indications

- Arthritis.
- Stiffness of spine.
- Gastro-intestinal disorders of stomach, intestine, liver, spleen and pancreas.
- Obesity of abdomen and thighs.
- Mental and physical fatigue.
- Diabetes.

ARDHA MATSYENDRASANA –I (LORD MATSYENDRA'S POSE)

Technique

- Sit with legs stretched in front.
- Bend right knee parallel to the floor, raise the hips, place foot horizontally under them and sit over it.
- Bend left knee vertically and place foot on outer side or right thigh with shin perpendicular to floor.
- Exhale and twist 90° to left, and bring right armpit over the left knee.
- Exhale and twist right arm around the left knee, and place it behind the back.
- Exhale and take left arm back, and grip the opposite hand.
- Turn head to left or right, and gaze at center of eyebrows or over the shoulder.
- Maintain the pose and breathe normally.
- Exhale and return to normal position.
- Repeat the pose sitting on the left foot and twisting to the right.

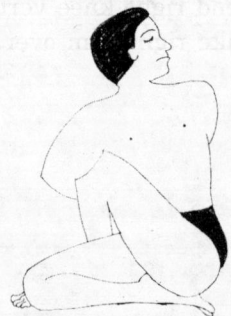

Figure 5.43: Adha-matsyendrasana-l

Advantages

- Tones complete spine.
- Massages abdominal and pelvic organs, especially the kidneys.
- Loosens all joints.
- Tones gonads and adrenal glands.
- Reduces fat around thighs, arms and waist.

Indications

- Spondylitis and backache.
- Genito-urinary bladder, uterus, ovary, testes and prostate.
- Gastro-intestinal disorders of liver, spleen and pancreas.
- Arthritis.
- Obesity around thighs, arm and waist.

JANU SIRSASANA (HEAD KNEE POSE)

Techniques

- Sit with legs straight and back erect.
- Bend right knee moving it to the right along the floor and place foot against left thigh as high as possible.
- Allow right knee to go backwards as much as possible to form an abuse angle between left and right thighs.
- Twist towards left with back straight to bring trunk in line with left leg.
- Inhale and raise arms up.
- Exhale and bend trunk and arms forward to the sides of foot of extended leg.
- Bend and widen elbows to allow trunk to move forwards.
- Allow head to rest on leg and keep extended chest on thigh.
- Maintain pose and breathe normally.
- Inhale and return to original position.
- Repeat pose with opposite leg straight.

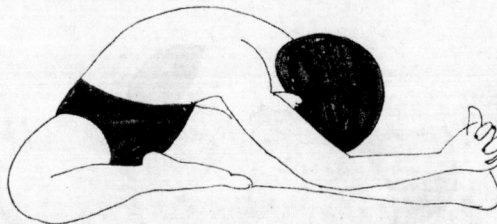

Figure 5.44: Janu Sirsasana

Advantages

- Tones complete spine.
- Tones abdominal organs.
- Relieves congestion in pelvic organs, prostate and gonads.
- Improve blood flow to pituitary, pineal, thyroid and parathyroid.
- Tones adrenals and islets of Langerhans.
- Soothes nerves and mind.
- Reduces stress and strain.
- Loosens joints of upper and lower extremities.
- Narrows the waist.

Indications

- Rigid and stiff spine.
- Indigestion and constipation.
- Liver, spleen and kidney disorders.
- Menstrual and sex gland disorders.
- Stress related diseases—hypertension, colitis, peptic ulcer, asthma, diabetes (with head resting on support).
- Mental or physical fatigue.
- Arthritis.
- Broad waist.

PASCIMOTTANASANA (BACK SPINE STRETCHING POSE)

Technique

- Sit with legs straight and back erect.
- Exhale and lean forwards and extending the arms from the shoulders to hold the toes.
- Exhale, bend forwards more by widening the elbows outwards.
- Bend and extend trunk further forwards and downwards from the hip towards legs, placing forehead on knees on legs or on support if unable to rest head on knees or legs.
- Hold toes or outer border of feet in the middle of the soles.

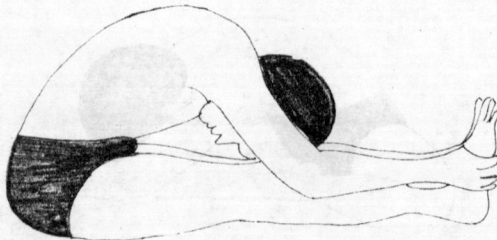

Figure 5.45: Pascirnottanasana

- Maintain the pose and breathe normally.
- Inhale and return to original pose.

Advantages

- Tones complete spine.
- Massages abdominal and pelvic organs.
- Improves digestion.
- Tones endocrine glands—adrenals, gonads, and islets of Langerhans.
- Removes mental and physical fatigue.
- Improves circulation of head and neck.
- Loosen all joints.

Indications

- Backache and arthritis.
- Gastro-intestinal disorders, constipation and dyspepsia,
- Diabetes, asthma and disorders of sex glands.
- Menstrual disorders.
- Stress related disorders—asthma, diabetes, peptic ulcer and colitis.
- Mental and physical fatigue.

Contraindication If pain is due to slipped disc or Sciatica.

MERU WAKRASANA (SPINAL TWIST POSE)

Technique

- Sit with legs stretched straight in front.
- Place the hands slightly behind and to the side of the buttocks.
- Finger should point backward.
- Put the left hand beside the right hand.

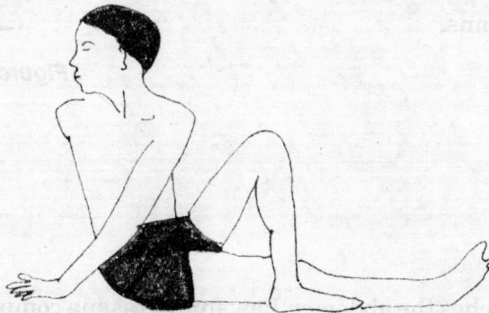

Figure 5.46: Meru Wakrasana

- Place the left foot outside the right knee. Move the right hand slightly backward.
- Twist the head and trunk as far as to the right.
- Exhale, return to the normal pose.
- Repeat with other side.

Advantages

- Twist the whole spine.
- Loosen all vertebrae.
- Massages all abdominal organs.

Indications

- Backache.
- Neckpain.
- Lumbago.
- Sciatica.

UTTAN PADASANA (RAISED FOOT POSE)

Technique

- Lie flat, leg together arms on side of the body.
- Inhale, raise the legs, keeping them straight and together.
- Arms should be relaxed on ground.
- Raise the feet up to 30-60 cms, not too high.
- Hold the legs simultaneously holding your breath.
- Exhale and slowly lower the feet.

Advantages

- Strength the abdominal muscles.
- Massages abdominal organs.
- Remove wind.

Figure 5.47: Uttan Padasana

Indications

- Obesity of abdomen
- Gastritis
- Constipation

Note—Uttan Padasana stretches the abdomen Pawanmuktasana compresses it. People suffering from flatulence or constipation. Practice one after another.

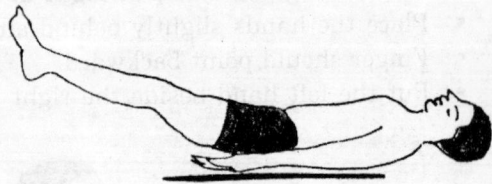

EKA PADA PRANAMASANA

Technique

- Stand upright with two feet together.
- Face forwards and gaze at a fixed point on the wall in front of your eyes.
- Bend one knee and place sole in contact with the thigh of other leg. Close to the perineum.
- Keep your hands in prayer position.
- Keep your eyes on the fixed point.
- Breathe normally, balance yourself in final pose.
- Repeat with other leg also.

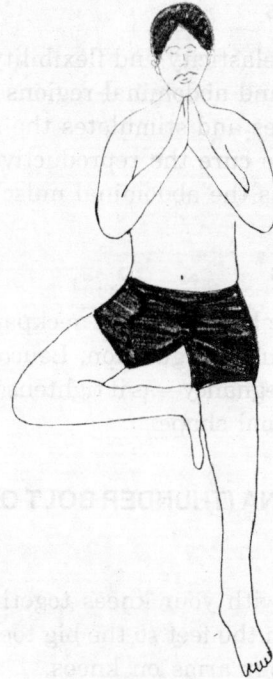

Advantages

- Bring nervous equilibrium
- Develop the sense of balance and co-ordination between different parts of the body.
- Develop concentration.

Indications

- In co-ordinated movements.
- Stress related disorders.

Figure 5.48: Eka Pada Pranamasana

MARJARIASANA (CAT STRETCH POSE)

Technique

- Knees on the ground.
- Lean forwards and place both hands flat on the floor in front of the knees (crawling)
- Arch your back upward while exhaling so that it forms a hump.
- Contract your abdomen to remove air as much as possible from lungs.
- Exhale, bring head between your arm facing towards thighs.
- Inhale, slowly press your back and raise your head.
- Spine should be concave as much as possible.
- Expand your abdomen, fill the lungs with maximum air.
- Exhale, raise your back upward & lower the head.
- Repeat the whole process again.

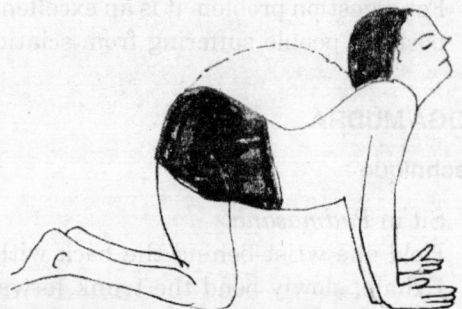

Figure 5.49: Marjariasana

Advantages

- Brings elasticity and flexibility of spine.
- Pelvic and abdominal regions are massaged.
- Stretches and stimulates the spinal nerves.
- Helps to cure the reproductive system disorders.
- Tightens the abdominal muscles.

Indications

- Chronic backache and neckpain.
- Menstrual irregulation, Leucorrhea.
- Post-pregnancy—as it tightens the abdominal muscles and encourage the abdomen to resume its normal shape.

VAJRASANA (THUNDER BOLT OR DIAMOND POSE)

Technique

- Kneel with your knees together.
- Position the feet so the big toes touches each other.
- Rest your arms on knees.
- Bring the buttocks downward onto the heels.
- Hold your head upright, neck and back straight.

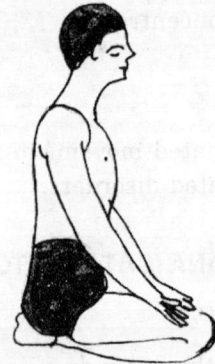

Advantages

- One of the few asanas which can be performed after food.
- Increase flexibility of ankles, knees.
- Helps in digestion.

Figure 5.50: Vajrasana

Indications

- For digestion problem it is an excellent meditative asana, and is the only perfect meditative posture, people suffering from sciatica and sacral infection.

YOGA MUDRA

Technique

- Sit in *Padmasana*.
- Hold one wrist behind the back with the other hand.
- Exhale, slowly bend the trunk forward until the forehead touches the ground.
- In the final position try to relax the whole body.
- Inhale, return to starting position.

Advantages

- Tones spine
- Massaging abdominal organs, endocrine glands.
- Alleviate various sexual disorders.
- Individual vertebrae are separated from each other, so it releases the pressure on spinal nerves.
- Stress disorders.
- Increases blood flow to head and neck.

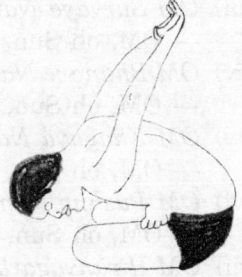

Figure 5.51: Yoga Mudra

Indications

- Stiffness of spine
- Gastro-intestinal disorders—dyspepsia, colitis, constipation.
- Liver and spleen disorders.
- Diabetes and asthma.
- Menstrual disorders.
- General tiredness and fatigue.
- Mental stress and strain.

SURYANAMASKAR

The sanskrit word 'Surya' means 'Sun' and 'Namaskar' means 'Salutation' or 'worship' so known as 'Salutation of the Sun'. Surya namaskar is a dynamic exercise. There are 12 phases of Kriyas (exercises). There are 12 mantras related to 12 cries also.

Basic Features

Surya Namaskar consists of five essential aspects. All of them should be done to gain the maximum result.

They are as follows –

1. **Physical Postures**: There are twelve physical postures, which correspond to the signs of the Zodiac.
2. **Breathing:** Each position is associated with inhalation, exhalation or retention of breathe. Detail of the correct relationship between movement and breathe are given later.
3. **Mantras:** Mantras are associated with each of the twelve positions of Surya namaskar. They are evocative sounds and through their power of vibration have subtle, but powerful and penetrating effects on the mind and body.

The mantras and their sequence are as follows –

i) *OM Mitraya Namah,* Mitra means friend.
   —Om, oh Sun, friend of the Universe, salutation to you. . .
ii) *OM Ravaye Namah,* Ravi means shining
   —OM, oh Sun, bringer of the motion in Universe, salutation to you.

iii) *OM Suryaya Namah.* Surya means beautiful light
— OM, oh Sun, giver of life, salutation to you.

iv) *OM Bhanave Namah,* Bhanu means brilliant
— OM, oh Sun, full of light, salutation to you.

v) *OM Khagaya Namah,* Khaga means who moves in the sky.
— OM, oh Sun, mover in the sky, salutation to you.

vi) *OM Pushne Namah,* Pushan means giver of strength
— OM, oh Sun, sustainer of world, salutation to you.

vii) *OM Hiranyagarbhaya Namah,* Hiranyagarbha means golden centered.
— Om, oh Sun, full of illumination salutation to you.

viii) *OM Marichaye Namah,* Marichi means lord of the dawn.
— OM, oh Sun, Lord of Rays, salutation to you.

ix) *OM Adityaya Namah,* Aditya means son of aditi.
— OM, oh Sun, savior of the world, salutation to you.

x) *OM Savitre Namah,* Savitre means beneficent.
— OM, oh Sun, creator of the world, salutation to you.

xi) *OM Arkaya Namah,* Arka means energy.
— OM, oh Sun, remover of impurity, salutation to you.

xii) *OM Bhaskaraya Namah,* Bhaskara means leading of enlightenment
— OM, oh Sun, maker of light, salutation to you.

4. **Awareness:** Every movement and breathing pattern should be well aware to the practitioner.

5. **Relaxation:** This is not strictly a part of Surya Namaskara. Any relaxation Technique can be adopted, but the best method is Shavasana. Rest of body and allow the heart beat and respiration to return to normal. It is also must to feel the mental peace and awareness.

TECHNIQUE, POSTURES AND BREATHING

POSITION ONE—PRANAMASANA TECHNIQUE (The Prayer Pose)

• Stand erect with the feet together
• Place your both palms together in prayer position in front of chest.
• Close the eye and relax the whole body.

Breathing—Breathe normally

Chant the mantra—*Om Mitraya Namah*

POSITION TWO—HASTA UTTANASANA (The Raised Arm Pose)

Technique

• Raise both arms above the head keeping hands separated by a shoulder's width.
• End of the movement bend (extend) head, arms and upper trunk backwards.

Breathing—Inhale while raising the arms.

Chant the mantra—'*Om Ravaye Namah*

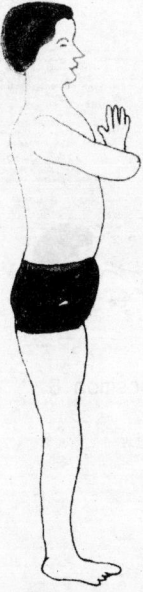

Figure 5.52a: Suryanamaskar—
position 1 and 12

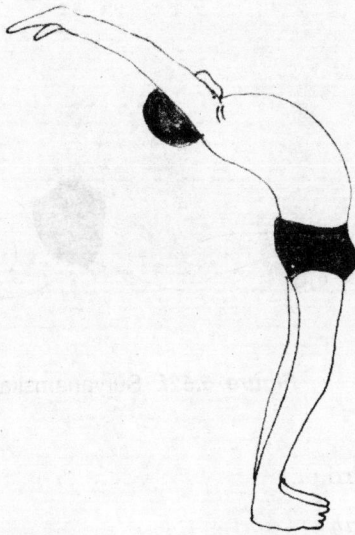

Figure 5.52b: Suryanamaskar—
position 2 and 11

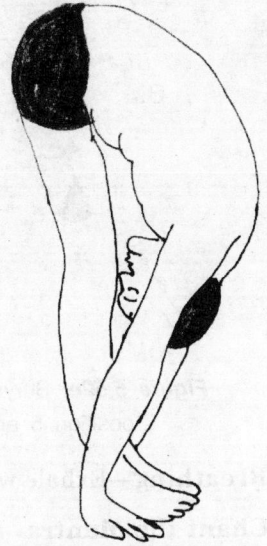

Figure 5.52c: Suryanamaskar—
position 3 and 10

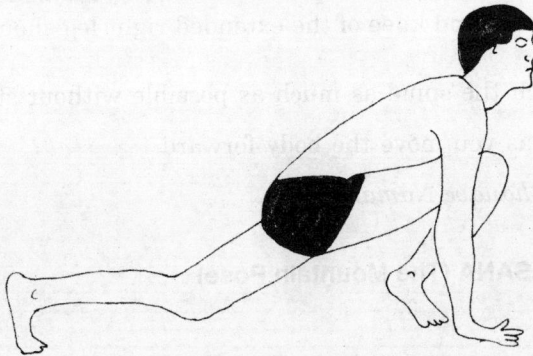

Figure 5.52d: Suryanamaskar—position 4 and 9

POSITION THREE—PADAHASTASANA (The Forward Bending Pose)

Technique

- Bend forward, place the palms on the ground either in front or side of the feet.
- Keep your knees straight.
- If possible, try to touch your knees with your forehead.
- Don't apply any force to attain the final position or give any jerky movement.

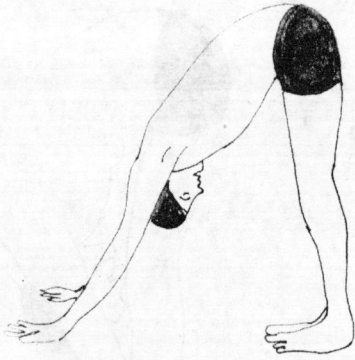

Figure 5.52e: Suryanamskar—
position 5 and 8

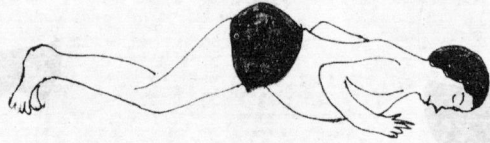

Figure 5.52f: Suryanamskar—position 6

Breathing—Exhale while bending forward.

Chant the Mantra—*Om Suryaya Namah*

POSITION FOUR—ASHWA SANCHALANASANA (The Equestrian Pose)

Technique

- Be in third position.
- Stretch the right leg backward as far as possible—Sit on your bended left leg.
- In the final position the toes and knee of the extended right leg should be in contact with the ground.
- Extend the neck and arch the spine as much as possible without straining.

Breathing—Inhale deeply as you move the body forward.

Chant the Mantra—*Om Bhanave Namah*

POSITION FIVE—PARVATASANA (The Mountain Pose)

Technique

- Raise your right knee.
- Simultaneously lower your head towards the floor.
- Stretch the left leg backward and place it with right leg.
- Raise the buttock as high as possible and lower the head between your two hand, so that you make a triangle.
- Legs should be straight.
- Try to press the heels of both feet towards the ground.

Breathing—Exhale while performing the movement.

Chant the Mantra—*Om Khagaya Namah.*

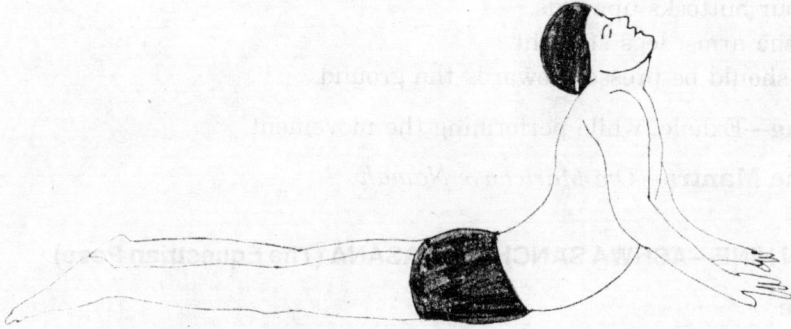

Figure 5.52g: Suryanamaskar—position 7

POSITION SIX—ASHTANGA NAMASKARA (Worship with Eight Points)

Technique

- This position is so called because in the final pose 8 points of the body are in contact with the ground—2 palms, 2 knees, 2 heels, chest and chin / head.
- Lower the body to the ground.
- Bend the legs and place your knees in contact with the floor.
- Bend the arms and lower the trunk towards the ground.
- Keep your chin or forehead on the floor.
- Keep the chest along with the floor.
- Finally raise the abdomen and hips slightly off the ground.

Breathing—Exhale, hold the breathe outside. Don't inhale.

Chant the Mantra—*Om Pushne Namah*

POSITION SEVEN—BHUJANGASANA (The Cobra Pose)

Technique

- Lower the hips to the ground.
- Straighten your arms.
- Take your head and back upward and backward till the navel level.

Breathing—Inhale while performing the movement.

Chant the Mantra—*Om Hiranyagarbhaya Namah*

POSITION EIGHT—PARVATASANA (The Mountain Pose)

Technique

- Same as position five.

- Lift your buttocks upwards.
- Keep the arms, legs straight.
- Heels should be pressed towards the ground.

Breathing—Exhale, while performing the movement.

Chant the Mantra—*Om Marichaye Namah*

POSITION NINE—ASHWA SANCHALANASANA (The Equestrian Pose)

Technique

- Same as position four.
- Stretch the other leg backward.
- Raise the head upward, arch the back downwards.
- Position of hands and foot must not be changed.

Breathing—Inhale.

Chant the Mantra—*Om Adityaya Namah*

POSITION TEN—PADAHASTASANA (Forward Bending Pose)

Technique

- This position is same as position three.
- Lower the head towards ground.
- Raise the buttock.
- Keep the right foot parallel to the left foot.
- Straighten the legs and try to touch the forehead to the knees.

Breathing—Exhale, as you move head towards the knees.

Chant the Mantra—*Om Savitre Namah*

POSITION ELEVEN—HASTA UTTANASANA (Raised Arm Pose)

Technique

- This position is same as position two.
- Straighten the whole body.
- Raise the arms over the head.
- Bend (extend) your back, neck, head and arms backward.

Breathing—Inhale.

Chant the Mantra—*Om Arkaya Namah*

POSITION TWELVE—PRANAMASANA (The Prayer Pose)

Technique

- This final pose is same as position one.
- Bring the palms together and hold them in front of chest.
- Relax the whole body.

Breathing—Exhale, breathe normally.

Chant the Mantra—*Om Bhaskaraya Namah*

Number of Rounds

The number of rounds depends on individual health and time available. Beginners should start with two rounds, adding one more round every second day. A person of good health should aim 12 rounds a day.

Contraindications / Limitations—There is absolutely no sex or age limitation. However ladies should not do it after fourth month of pregnancy, it can be continued after childbirth.

Ladies should not do during menstruation as a precautionary measure.

People with sciatica, slipped disc, high blood pressure, coronary heart disease should not do Suryanamaskar.

Benefits—It exercises the entire body. It is an intelligent exercise that influences the health of the whole body.

The body consists of various systems and organs, which interrelate and co-ordinate with each other to give the best possible health and efficiency. Let us discuss some of the main systems in the body and how they are benefited.

- **Digestive system**—The abdominal organs and stomach are alternately stretched and compressed. This gives massage to the internal organs and ensures that they function correctly. Many diseases of the digestive system can be prevented and removed by the regular practice of Suryanamaskar.
- **Excretory system**—Suryanamaskar stimulates the peristalsis and helps to remove any tendency towards constipation. It gives gentle massage to kidney, increases the blood supply, as well as speed up the circulation throughout the body. For best result one should drink plenty of clean, fresh water before practice. Suryanamaskar results in increased perspiration and encourages the elimination of toxins from the body, helping to prevent skin ailments.
- **Circulatory system**—It increases the heartbeat and working of the whole circulatory system, helps to eliminate waste materials from the body, increases nutrition to the cell.

  Lymphatic system is also speeded up. This system is not important in protecting the body against infection. Suryanamaskar, by increasing the circulatory and removal of poisonous bacteria, directly aids the lymphatic system to work more efficiently in its fight against illness.
- **Respiratory system**—Suryanamaskar, when done correctly, accentuates the exchange of air to and from the lungs, opens and expands the intricate alveoli or air sacs of the lung,

tissue and exercises the muscles of the surrounding chest region. Body and brain are revitalized by the extra supply of oxygen.

- **Endocrinal system**—This system plays an important role in our good health. It consists of large number of different hormones, which plays an important role in maintaining good health. Even the slightest imbalance can cause some form of disease. A well known example is diabetes.

    Suryanamaskar harmonizes this system helping to remove any irregularities by directly massaging the relevant glands and improving their blood flow. Imbalance of the endocrine system is often caused by mental tension, which can be very much reduced by Suryanamaskar.

- **Nervous system**—The multitudes of nervous connections throughout the body are gently stretched, massaged and stimulated. The nerves are the intermediaries. If the nerves are unhealthy then the functioning of associated organ must suffer. Suryanamaskar tones up these nerves and simultaneously awakens the associated brain centers. One feels more alive after a few rounds of this exercise.

- **Muscles and skeleton**—Suryanamaskar exercises all the main muscles and joints in the body. It is an excellent method of loosening the body and joints.

- **Subtle influence**—Suryanamaskar can give additional and more benefits beyond the physical. If you are totally involved with the mantras, the breathing and the movements, it will induce peace of mind. It is therefore a very useful exercise in reducing emotional conflict, neurosis and stress. This purify the heart and mind. Suryanamaskar is an excellent practice with which to start the day. It helps to prepare you in every way to face the oncoming day with physical and mental strength and confidence.

SAVASANA (The Corpse Pose)

This is also known as Mitrasana (Dead Man's Pose).

Technique

- Lie flat on back in spine with center of forehead, chin, sternum, navel and pubis in one line.
- Keep arms slightly away from the side of the body, palms facing upwards.
- Legs should be straight and slightly separated.
- Close your eyes.
- Breathe normally with full awareness.
- Try to feel different parts of your body in contact with the floor.
- If the muscles of the buttocks' are pulled together, then release them.
- Now try to feel the contact between the ground and the right heel for a few seconds.
- Repeat the same with left heel.
- Now feel the contact between the floor and the right arm, right hand, left arm, left hand, the middle of the back, each shoulder blade, back of the head and finally the whole body.
- Spend a few seconds at each point.

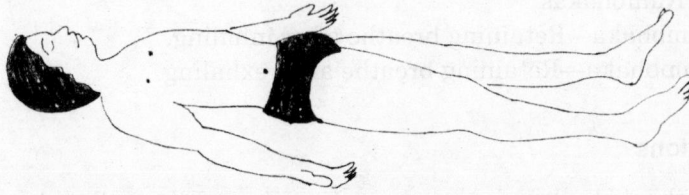

Figure 5.53: Savasana

- Now try to release the tension from right hand, left hand, both legs, each joint and finally the whole body.
- Throughout the practice your worries or problems may keep appearing. Don't suppress the thoughts if they occur, merely continue to direct your attention to the systematic relaxation of the different parts of the body and try to breathe relaxed and normally.
- You will attend a wonderful relaxed state physically and mentally. When you finish the practice, gently move and clench your hands, move feet and slowly open your eyes.

Note—During the asana, don't go to sleep and be fully aware of the breathe and the relaxed state of body and mind.

Advantages

- Reduces physical, mental and emotional stress, strain and fatigue of all kind.
- Gives total relaxation to body.
- Soothes nerves and mind.
- Reduces basal metabolic rate, pulse and blood pressure.

Indications

- Physical and mental fatigue and tension.
- Insomnia, anxiety, neurosis and phobia.
- Stress related disease, asthma, diabetes, peptic ulcer, colitis and angina pectoris.
- High blood pressure, tachycardia and hyper thyroidism.

PRANAYAMA

There are two words in *Pranayama*, Prana and Ayam. The meaning of 'Prana' is life force oxygen and breathe. 'Ayam' means to lengthen, to spread, to control and to retain. Thus Pranayam means 'Lengthening, Controlling and Retaining the life force'.

Breathe in, breathe out and control breathing—the three processes together is known as *Pranayama*.

- Rechaka—The process of exhaling or breathing out.
- Puraka—The process of inhaling or breathing in.
- Kumbhaka—The process of retaining breathe.

There are two Kumbhakas:
- Internal Kumbhaka—Retaining breathe after inhaling.
- External Kumbhaka—Retaining breathe after exhaling.

Hints and Cautions

- Pranayama should be done in an open space or in a well-ventilated room, free from insects, while sitting on a blanket, a carpet or mat.
- Place should be clean, quiet and free from foul smell or smoke.
- Evacuate the bowel and empty the bladder before starting Pranayama.
- Preferably Pranayama should be practised in empty stomach but if it is difficult, tea, coffee can be taken. At least five to six hours to elapse after a meal before practicing Pranayama.
- The best time to practice is the early morning and after sunset.
- Clothing should be light and loose.
- For doing Pranayama, best asana—*Padmasana, Siddhasana, Virasana, Sukhasana*—can also be adopted for doing Pranayama.
- During practice no strain should be felt in the facial muscle, eyes and ears or in the neck muscle, shoulder, arms, thighs and the feet.
- Keep the eyes closed throughout.
- The waist, back and neck should remain erect during the practice of Pranayama.
- Try to achieve an even ratio in inhalation (Puraka) and exhalation (Rechaka). For example, if one is for 5 seconds during a given continuous cycle, the other should be for the same time.

The Method of Closing the Nostrils (NASAGRA MUDRA)

- Breathe through the nostril is controlled by fingers of one hand held in front of the face.
- Hold the right hand in front of the face.
- Place the tip of the second (index) and third finger so that they rest on the forehead at the eyebrow center.
- In this position, the thumb should be beside the right nostril and the ring finger (fourth) beside the left nostril.
- The airflow through the left nostril is controlled by ring finger.
- The elbow of right arm should be near to chest.

NADI SHODHANA PRANAYAMA

Posture Technique

- Sit in *Padmasana, Sukhasana* or *Vajrasana* can also be adopted.
- Relax your whole body.
- Hold the spine upright.
- Place the left hand on the right hand.

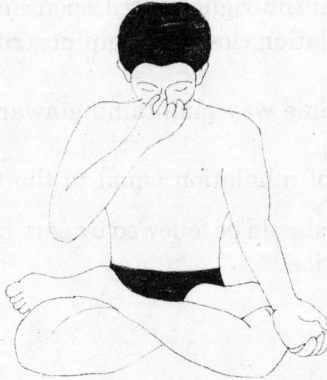

Figure 5.54: Nadi Shodhana Pranayama

- Do nasagra mudra with right hand.
- Close the eye.

Breathing Technique (Part 1)

- Close the right nostril with the thumb.
- Slowly inhale through the left nostril.
- Simultaneously mentally count 1-2-3 each interval being about 1 second.
- Exhale through the left nostril only. Again count mentally.
- Try to make the length of exhalation twice as long as inhalation.
- Do 5-10 rounds through the left nostril.
- Then close the left nostril using the fourth finger, open the right nostril and do the same as much as you have done with left nostril.
- Be aware of the breathe and the mental counting throughout the practice.

Breathing Technique (Part 2)

- Sit in *Padmasana* or any suitable above mentioned asanas.
- Be calm and relax whole body.
- Close your eyes.
- Be in nasgara mudra.
- Close the right nostril with the thumb.
- Inhale through the left nostril.
- Breathe as deeply as possible utilizing the abdomen and chest to fill the lungs to the maximum with air.
- At the end of inhalation close the left nostril.
- Open the right nostril and exhale.
- Exhale slowly to the maximum.

- At the end of exhalation keep the right nostril open and then slowly inhale.
- After completing the full inhalation close the right nostril, open the left nostril and exhale.
- This is one round.
- Do few more rounds in the same way maintaining awareness of the breathe and mental counting.
- Try to balance the duration of inhalation equal to the time of exhalation.

Sequence—Nadi Shodhana part 2 should be followed by part 1. They should be done after asanas and before relaxation or meditation.

Precautions

- Avoid retention of breathe (Kumbhaka) in problems of ears, eyes, heart, lungs and brain.
- If there is a sign of discomfort reduce the duration of inhalation and exhalation.

Benefits

- Improves oxygenation of blood and tissues.
- Improves function of all organs and systems.
- Balances automatic nervous system.
- Calms nerves and mind.
- Reduces stress and strain.
- Improves immune system.
- Stabilizes cardio-respiratory system.
- It helps to remove congestion or blockage of the nadis and thereby allows the free flow of Prana.

Indications

- Respiratory disorders—Asthma, Bronchitis, Respiratory tract infection, Chronic coughs and cold (in all without retention of breath).
- Stress related disorders—Vasomotor, rhinits, peptic ulcers, diabetes and Colitis.
- Physical or mental tension.
- Cardiovascular disorders—Angina pectoris, Cardiac arrhythmias, Hypertension (without retention of breath).
- Convalescence from various disease.
- Insomnia, poor memory, concentration (without retention of breath).

SHEETALI PRANAYAMA (Cooling practice)

The sanskrit word Sheetali means 'Cooling' or 'relaxing'. It cools down the body and relaxes the mind.

Rolling of Tongue

During inhalation the tongue has to be rolled.

Roll the tongue so that both side curl upwards and inwards with edges almost meeting each other. The end of the tongue should protrude outside the mouth. The rolled tongue forms a tube through which one inhales.

Technique

- Sit in *Padmasana*
- Close the eye and relax the whole body.
- Be aware of breathing
- Roll the tongue.
- Slowly inhale through the tube formed by rolled tongue.
- Hold the breathe.
- Withdraw the tongue and close the mouth.
- Retain breathe.
- Exhale slowly through the nose.
- Be aware of breathe flow and relax.
- This is one round.
- Start with 3-4 times go up to 15-20 times.

Advantages

- Cools down the body and mind.
- Soothe away mental tension
- Purify blood.
- Improves bile digestion.
- Regulates bile flow.
- Revitalizes skin and eyes.

Indications

- High blood pressure.
- Digestive disorders.
- Dryness of mouth.
- Tonsillitis
- Psychosomatic diseases.

Note: In general breathing inhalation is done through nose, but in this it is done by mouth so

  (a) Do not practice in a dirty, polluted atmosphere
  (b) Avoid practicing in excessively cold weather.

TRATAKA

The word 'TRATAKA' means 'Steady gazing'. The practice of trataka involves gazing at a point or object without blinking the eyes and in turn the mind on one point to the exclusion of all others.

Choice of object can be anything such as a candle flame, a cross, AUM symbol, A flower, Nose tip, Yin and Yang symbol, Crystal, Statuette of Buddha, Christ, a fixed point and many more things.

But candle flame is the best choice for the beginners.

Posture

Sit in *Padmasana, Siddhasana* or any most comfortable sitting position, even sitting on a chair. Sit relaxed, breathe normally.

Position of Object

Place the desired object (a candle) in horizontal level as eyes and at an arm's length (2 meters) from the eyes.

Technique

- Light the candle and place it on a small bench, so that the flame is at eye level when you sit on the floor.
- Sit on floor and adjust your position so that the candle is at an arm's length.
- Keep the spine erect.
- Close the eyes and relax the whole body.
- Open your eyes.
- Gaze intently at the flame, directing your attention particularly to the top of the flame.
- Don't look any thing else but flame and wick.
- Try not to blink your eyelids or move your eyeballs.
- Don't strain the eyes.
- If you feel pain in eye, blink it.
- Initially continue gazing for about 2-3 minutes.
- Close your eyes.
- Try to visualise the after-image of the candle flame in front of your closed eyes.
- When the image begins to fade open your eyes and again gaze at the candle flame and wick.
- Continue this outer gazing for about 2 or 3 minutes.
- Once again close the eyes and gaze at the inner image.
- Continue to repeat inner trataka and outer trataka one after the other.
- Before finishing close the eyes and watch the dark space in front of your closed eyes.
- Open your eyes and relax.

Advantages

- It develops the power of concentration.
- Induces peace of mind.
- Power of memory improves.
- Eyesight improves
- Strengths eye muscles.

Indications

- Lack of concentration
- Stress, strain, nervous, tension
- Sleep related disorders—Insomnia.
- Eye-disorders.

SECTION 2
STRESS MANAGEMENT

chapter six

What is Stress?

Stress is a everyday fact of life. It is global and today it exists as an epidemic.

Modern man, in spite of his current level of progress and advancement, is yet to conquer stress. In today's high pressure world, the stresses and strains of modern living can become increasingly hard to bear. Stress is something which cannot be avoided.

Though we do differ in the extent to which we are stressed and the way in which we react to it, the fact remains that all of us are affected by it in one way or the other.

In a study conducted by Harnet School of Public Health predicted the global burden of disease and injury in the year 2020, it would appear that stress killing the people as compared with infected diseases will be more. So stress management is going to be major future concern for all those who deal with human health.

In simple terms, stress is a reaction or response to any kind of change. It is the physical and emotional response to situation, which are perceived as frightening, confusing, exciting or tiring. It not only gets precipitated by external demands, but can also be generated from within by our hopes, fears, expectations and beliefs. It acts like a signal for the mind and body to get prepared for any eventuality.

STRESS—GOOD OR BAD

All stress is not bad. We sometimes hear people saying 'I work for better under pressure or tension'. There are other class of people who endlessly crib about work pressure, mounting price, water shortage, what we need is a balance.

Stress can be positive or negative. We always think of negative events or situations as the cause of stress. Some positive changes like, marriage, getting a new and better job, winning a match, Good results or becoming a parent prove to be stressful due to increased pressure and responsibilities. But since they are associated with positive feelings of pleasure, confidence, excitement, happiness, love and joy, they actually increase our resistance to stress. On the other hand negative situations such as illness, death, difficulty at the workplace, low income are all associated with negative feeling such as sadness, dissatisfaction, irritation. These feelings lower our resistance to stress and make us more prone to mental disturbances and diseases.

Stress is not only desirable but essential to life. A certain amount of stress is essential for normal health.

'Complete freedom from stress is death'. Some stress is required to stimulate us to do day-to-day task. In today's competitive world, its presence is more important. It is not just a pathological symptom, it is an essential feature of the mechanism which drives people.

Any event or situation which is perceived as threatening demands active coping.

When feeling of stress override all the other emotions and the 'good' stress get depressed, we feel tense, worried, anxious. This is the time when stress becomes 'bad' and need to be managed. It is better to manage stress responses rather than try to remove them.

chapter seven

Stressors: Factors that Produce Stress

Stressors are the pressures that induce the stress. Stress has many meanings but most of us think, stress as the demands of life. These demands are called 'Stressors' and the actual wear and tear on our bodies is the stress.

These stressors or demands of life can come from people and events around us, as well as from our inner thoughts and struggles.

Stressors: Where does stress come from?

As we have defined stressors as the external demand of life or the internal attitude or thoughts. It can include traffic jam, divorce, death or the angry boss, pollution all-around.

We can keep them in different categories.

DOMESTIC STRESSORS

Interactions with family members can be stressful. The marriage was once a strong, supportive force that could help family members cope with other stressors. Now nearly 20-30% of all marriages end in divorce. The birth of a child places new demands for adaptation on a family. Some examples of domestic stressors are as below:

Marriage

- Difference in mutual interests.
- Recurrent financial problem.
- Unfaithfulness.
- Sexual difficulties leading to frustration.
- Illness of spouse.
- Prolonged separation.
- Conflicting careers.

Children

- Sick child left with permanent impairment
- Handicapped child
- Disobedient child
- Poor academic performance
- Bad behavior at school
- Drinking habits or with drug problem

Other Domestic and Social Stressors

- Single parent family
- Aging parents
- Demanding in-laws
- Unplanned pregnancy
- Difficult neighbors

OCCUPATIONAL OR WORK STRESSORS

A major part of our life spend at our workplace. Work plays an important role in determining one's identity.

The term job stress brings like job dissatisfaction, work overload, uncertainty. Some examples of work stressors are:

Occupational Stressors

- Change in new job requires new skills
- Low salary
- Inadequate rewards
- Unclear goal
- Hostile customers
- Incompetent co-workers
- New management style
- Frequent night shifts
- Insufficient time to do job properly
- Poor prospects

Physical and Environmental Stressors

- Noisy surroundings
- Poor lighting
- Toxic fumes
- Precision work causing eye strain
- Poor ventilation
- Unhygienic condition

Psychological Stressors

- Office politics
- Isolated environment
- Sexual harassment
- Rude people
- Bullies
- Hostile atmosphere

PHOBIC STRESSORS

Many people have exaggerated fears of certain animals, places, objects, is called phobias. Some of them are:

- Claustrophobia (Small enclosed space)
- Acrophobia (Height)
- Aquaphobia (Water)
- School phobia
- Ergasiophobia (work)
- Cibophobia (food)
- Onomatophobia (names or terms)

DISEASE AND PAIN STRESSORS

Disease stressors are those which we experience as a result of long or short term disorders. For example, some people are born with a predisposition to develop headaches, arthritis, ulcers, high blood pressure, diabetes, multiple sclerosis.

These conditions may or may not be caused by stress, but can be aggravated by stress. Pain stressors are the aches and pains of new and old injuries, accidents or disease.

ECONOMIC, POLITICAL AND SOCIAL STRESSORS

Economic

- Slow economic growth
- Energy crisis
- Increase imports
- Consumer boom
- Unemployment
- Exorbitant property prices

Political

- Income-tax
- Bureaucracy
- Lack of leadership
- Insurgency or terrorism
- Corrupt government

Social

- Class discrimination
- Over population
- Social isolation
- Housing shortage
- Social outcast
- Communal tension

chapter eight

How Our Body Responds to Stress?

There are four general reactions to stress, the normal in which the alert is followed by an action of defense. The neurotic in which the alert or anxiety is so great that the defense becomes ineffective, the psychotic in which the alarm may be misinterpreted or even ignored and the psychosomatic in which the defense by the mind fails and the alert is transmitted into the bodily systems causing changes in body tissues.

Thus, prolonged alertness and tension can produce physiological disorders, involving specific body organs, ranging from minor ailments like tension, headache, migraine and backache while triggering off asthma, eczema, arthritis, palpitation, indigestion, diarrhoea, constipation and disturbed sleep.

Following are common stress disorders:

High blood pressure   Hypertension or high blood pressure is directly related to the stress. Uncontrolled high blood pressure can strain the heart and contribute to the hardening of blood vessels, which causes premature heart attacks, neurological problems and other diseases of the blood vessels.

Angina pectoris is another commonly seen problem which is characterised by tight gripping pain in the centre of the chest, often radiating to the left, or sometimes, to both arms, neck, throat or jaw.

HEART ATTACK

Cigarette smoking, excessive drinking and stress hormones are known to increase the stickiness of the blood cells making them prone to make thrombus which is the major cause of heart attack. Blood supply through that part of the blood vessel is completely cut off. That part of the heart muscle supplied by the blocked section dies. Chest pain is similar to angina but occurs even at rest and lasts longer.

PALPITATION AND CHEST DISCOMFORT

Palpitation increases the heartbeats. The normal heartbeat rate ranges between 60 to 80 beats per minutes. During physical or mental exertion, the rate rise to 150 or even 200 beats per minutes. Stress, anxiety, excessive alcohol and smoking frequently cause palpitation.

MIGRAINE AND TENSION HEADACHE

When the muscle around the head remains tense for sometime, it may lead to tension headache. Migraine is different from tension headache.

CHRONIC FATIGUE

A constant feeling of tiredness or fatigue, is the commonest symptom of stress.

Fatigue can develop due to physical or mental, exertion. Stress, whether physical, mental or emotional, drains up of energy. Fatigue causes disturbances in our mood and concentration and reduces our capacity to work.

ULCER

Stress causes increased secretion of acid which causes hyperacidity, peptic activity derived from pepsinogen is a major cause of ulcer production. It suppresses the secretion of a surface mucus layer by epithelial cells. Regenerative capacity of mucosal epithilial cells is reduced. So inner lining of the stomach gets eroded. Most prominent symptom is pain.

DIABETES MELLITUS

Stress aggravates latent diabetes, it does not cause it. In diabetes rigid diet and medicines are followed, it may produce stress which is often beyond the patient's adapting and coping capacities. Physical and emotional stress can cause a worsening of blood sugar control.

ASTHMA

In an asthmatic attack, the small bronchial tubes which carry the air in and out of the lungs get narrowed. As a result, it becomes difficult to get enough air and the affected person becomes short of breath and starts coughing. Person starts wheezing. Stress can trigger off a wheezing attack. Stress may or may not be directly related to the cause of the disorder, but its presence over a prolonged period of time is related to worsening of the condition.

IRRITABLE BOWEL SYNDROME

In this condition, the person experiences lower abdomen pain, diarrhoea, alternating with constipation, increased frequency of stool with a feeling that the bowel has not been completely emptied. Stress is often an exacerbating factor.

COLD AND COUGHS

Susceptibility to cold is directly related to the intensity of stress. Stress reduces the effectiveness of our immune system. Thus highly stressed people have a tendency to suffer more frequently from cold and symptom tend to last longer.

DEPRESSION

The effect of long-term stress can be devastating. Under long-term stress our personalities may change. We may suffer from depression, feel hopeless, helpless and overwhelmingly bleak and burdensome life.

BACKACHE

In stressful condition, physical discomfort may become so magnified, as to be incapacitating. Thus, a chronic domestic worry, job dissatisfaction, interpersonal problems, prolong work may severely aggravate it.

Over stress can harm us. Thus, it is important to recognize its early signs and symptoms as timely intervention can prevent the developing of serious health hazards whether physical, mental or psychosomatic.

chapter nine

Coping with Stress

Stress whether good or bad, is all pervading facet of life.

Coping with stress means the ways and means you adopt to keep stress at manageable level, bring about certain changes in yourself, so that you perceive the stressor as not so threatening, or find ways to convert it into a motivating or driving force.

NEGATIVE COPING METHODS

Coping of stress can be negative or positive. Let's first talk about negative coping. By negative coping we mean those attempts to manage or control stress, which at that time seems to be worthwhile efforts, but in reality only further add to the stress level in imperceptible ways. Some of these negative coping techniques initially combat the immediate effects of the stressful event or situation, giving a false sense of relief and comfort and thus making you resort to these methods of coping again. These methods have a cumulative negative effect on your body and mind and you may feel their damaging effects when it is too late to change this coping pattern. For example, alcohol is a selective and progressive depressant of brain functions. Though initially a small quantity may lift your inhibitions and make you feel confident. Once the tranquilizing effect wears off, an upsurge of anxiety and tension erupts. Excessive drinking can cause physical diseases, memory disturbances, brain damage, and induce aggression or anger. Which finally leads to breakdown of family life and greater amount of stress which goes beyond coping.

Few unhealthy habits like drinking, smoking, eating too much or too little food, resorting to drugs or tranquilizers, drinking too much coffee, sleeping too much, increases susceptibility to stress.

POSITIVE COPING METHODS

Certain healthy habits on the other hand, can actually help reduce stress and its effects on both the body and the mind.

Nutrition

"What we eat we are'. What and how we eat determines how healthy we can be able to prevent disease. Some believe that nutritious balanced diet, eaten at regular, fixed hours is a good antidote to the tensions of daily living. High dose of vitamin supplements, especially Vitamin

B complex, C and E protect against stress and strain by giving a boost to the immune system and increasing resistance levels. Natural diet rich in vitamins and minerals essentially does the same, keeps the body healthy and strong to cope with the ravages of stress.

Relationship

Stress and its effects can be offset by turning them positively in social relationship. Sometimes stressful events can lead to meaningful relationships with others. It can bring you closer to a relative or friend in the process of sharing your burdens or problems.

Exercise

Exercise is an effective way to deal with the tensions of modern life. A vigorous physical activity, workout, or a sport reduces the stress and eventually returns to a balanced state of mind and body. Regular exercise, workout or a sport may relieve from stress and strain, leaving you fresh, alert and rejuvenated.

Sometimes to break the boring and monotonous routine, which produces a different kind of stress, we can go for some adventurous leisure pursuits such as mountaineering, sailing, car racing and many more. These are examples of healthy coping methods to deal with boredom and stessors.

Diversion

These include films, music, television. These are temporary diversions or 'escape' from the pressing problems of daily living. There activities provide a source of joy and entertainment with safe outlet to resolve your inner tension. But diversion is temporary solution, though the approach is positive. Their benefits are short-term and short-lived.

Removal

Another way to relieve stress is getting away for brief periods of time to resorts in mountains, beaches or long tour. These periodic retreats provide the much needed change of environment with rest, a relaxed atmosphere, better eating and sleeping habits that restore the mind and body and recharge you to face the stress better when you get back.

For others, removal of stress lies in some form of spiritual commitment by way of gurus, godmen, meditation. So being positive in thinking and in action, may make your stress more bearable and may even lead to mastery over what appears unbearable.

chapter ten

Mental Techniques to Combat Stress

How can we relax and learn to do it well? Relaxation techniques start by taking your consciousness away from emotionally-charged thoughts and directing it to activities that are emotionally neutral such as the awareness of your breath or different parts of your body.

BREATHING

Breathing is essential to life. It is automatic and usually involuntary, but is also unique that it can be controlled by deliberate effort. It can affect our emotional and physical feelings. Thus, proper breathing habits are essential for good mental and physical health.

Types of Breathing

There are basically two types of breathing (i) Chest breathing and (ii) Abdominal breathing.

Chest breathing is characterized by an upward, outward, movement of the chest wall. The breath is shallow, and unsteady. It is usually seen when the body is aroused by certain challenging or stressful situations. There is direct relationship between the mind and breathing. Until and unless this shallow and unsteady breathing is replaced by deep and even abdominal breathing, the body will continue to be in a state of constant arousal and tension.

Abdominal breathing is also called diaphragmatic breathing, since it involves the diaphragm. When we inhale, diaphragm contracts and pushes downwards. This relaxes the abdominal muscles. While breathing out, the diaphragm relaxes and the abdominal muscles contract to expel the impure air. It is the most efficient type of breathing, because it enhances greater expansion and ventilation of the lungs. It also improves circulation. When we are calm and relaxed, our breathing is abdominal and due to the direct relationship between the mind and breathing, practicing abdominal breathing leads to mental as well as physical relaxation.

Breathing exercise can help in reducing anxiety, depression, irritability, muscle tension and fatigue. A breathing exercise can be learned in a matter of minutes and some immediate benefits experienced, but its profounder effects may not be fully apparent until months of persistent practice have passed.

A Simple Deep Breathing Exercise

Concentrate on your breathing several times during the day. It could be done anywhere, anytime. Close your eyes, take a deep breath. Inhale through your nose. Feel the energy coming in and revitalizing your body. Breath out through your mouth, making a quiet, relaxing, whooshing sound like the wind as you gently blow out. Try to concentrate over your breathing. Continue to take long, slow, deep breaths which raise and lower your abdomen.

Continue deep breathing for about five to ten minutes at a time. Feel relaxed, extend the time as per your wish. At the end of each deep breathing session, scan your body for tension and compare the tension with that tension which you experienced when you started. When you have learned to relax yourself using deep breathing, practice it whenever you feel yourself getting tense, angry or worked up and breathe away to a state of almost instant relaxation.

Progressive Relaxation Technique

Nothing perhaps has been so grossly misunderstood as the art of relaxation. It does not mean lying around and doing nothing. Relaxation really means rest after effort, more truly, conscious rest after conscious effort.

The three major forms of current relaxation practice—meditation, progressive relaxation and autogenics.

Progressive Relaxation

Progressive relaxation, which is one of the most commonly used technique was developed by Edmond Jacobson. According to him, the body responds to anxiety provoking thought and events with muscle tension. This bodily tension increases the subjective experience of anxiety. This physiology or bodily tension is reduced by muscular relaxation, which thereby reduces anxiety.

Indications

It gives excellent results in the treatment of muscular tension, anxiety, insomnia, fatigue, irritable bowels, muscle spasm, neck and back pain, high blood pressure, mild phobias and stuttering.

Technique of Progressive Muscular Relaxation

In progressive relaxation, you first tense and then relax each group of muscle. This helps focus attention on the feeling of tension in the body. The higher your awareness of the tension, the easier it is to control it.

Squeeze a particular muscle group firmly and maintain tension for five to ten seconds. Release the tension quickly so that muscles relax immediately and you are easily able to differentiate between relaxation and tension.

It is important to remember that only one specific muscle group at a time should be tensed, the rest of the body should remain in relaxed position.

By full attention to whatever you are doing in the exercise—relaxing or tensing.

Position

Sitting in a comfortable armchair with a high back, or lying down on a flat surface on a thin mattress. Clothing should be loose and comfortable. Close your eyes.

Step 1   Take a comfortable position and relax. Now clench your right fist tighter and tighter. Keep it clenched and notice the tension in your fist, hand and forearm, now relax. Feel the looseness in your right hand and note the contrast with its earlier tension. Repeat this procedure with your right fist remaining constantly aware of the state of tension and it's easing. Repeat with your left fist, then both fists together.

Step 2   Now bend your elbow and tense your biceps. Tense them as hard as you can and feel the tightness. Relax and straighten out your arms. Let the relaxation develop and feel the difference.

Step 3   Next, wrinkle your forehead as much as you can. Let it relax. Imagine your entire forehead and scalp becoming smooth and at rest. Allow your brow to relax. Close your eyes tightly, feel the tension and slowly let them relax.

Step 4   Now tighten your jaw by pressing the teeth together. Feel the tension and then slowly relax your jaw. When the jaw is relaxed, your lips will be slightly parted. Observe the contrast between tension and relaxation. Now press your tongue almost against the roof of your mouth. Feel the ache in the back of your mouth. Relax. Press your lips now. Relax your lips. Notice that your forehead, scalp, tongue and lips are now relaxed.

Step 5   Press your head back as far as it can comfortably go and observe the tension in your neck. Roll it to the right, then to the left and feel the changing locus of stress. Straighten your head and bring it forward. Press your chin against your chest. Feel the tension in your throat and in the back of your neck. Relax, allowing your head to return to a comfortable position. Allow the feeling of relaxation to deepen.

Step 6   Now shrug your shoulders. Keep the tension as you hunch your head down between your shoulders. Relax your shoulders.

Step 7   Let your entire body relax. Feel the comfort and the heaviness. Breathe in and fill your lungs comfortably. Hold your breath. Observe the tension. Now exhale, let your chest loosen, and the air hiss out. Continue relaxing, letting your breath come freely and gently. Repeat this several times and feel the tension draining from your body as you exhale. Next tighten your stomach. Breathe deeply. Hold and relax. Observe the contrast to the earlier tension as you exhale. Now arch your back without straining. Keep the rest of your body as relaxed as possible. Focus on the tension in your lower back. Now relax deeper and deeper.

Step 8   Tighten your buttocks and thighs. Press your thighs by pressing down your heels as hard as you can. Relax and feel the difference. Now curl your toes downwards, tensing your calves. Feel the tension, then relax. Now bend your toes toward your face, creating tension in your shins. Relax again.

Step 9   Feel the heaviness in your lower body as the sense of relaxation deepens. Relax your feet, ankles, calves, shins, knees, thighs, and buttocks. Now let the relaxation spread to your stomach, lower back and chest. Let go more and more. Experience the relaxation deepening in your shoulders, arms and hands deeper and deeper. Notice the feeling of looseness and relaxation in your neck, jaws and facial muscle.

Step 10   You are completely relaxed now. Keep lying down. Don't move. Keep your eyes closed and enjoy this peaceful experience. After a few second count slowly from one to five then from five to one. Now slowly open your eyes. Turn over on your side. Keep lying down for a few more minutes, then slowly sit up with the support of your arm.

It is always advisable to get up very slowly after a tension relaxation exercise, so that body can gradually readjust to the pressure of work. If you get up too quickly, you may feel dizzy, light headed or even nauseated, due to sudden load on the bodily system, which has slowed down in the process of relaxation.

AUTOGENIC RELAXATION TECHNIQUE

Autogenic means self-generating. It was developed by Johannes Shultz. It is a systematic programme that teaches the body and mind to respond quickly and effectively to verbal commands to relax and return to a balanced, normal state. It consists of a series of phrases, which we can repeat to ourselves as self or auto suggestions.

Shultz's verbal formula falls into three kinds of exercises—the standard exercises concentrate on the body, the meditative exercises focus on the mind and some special exercises that have been developed to normalize specific problems.

The first standard exercise focuses on the theme of heaviness. The suggestions of heaviness in the limbs actually leads to the feeling of heaviness associated with relaxation.

The second exercise brings about peripheral vasodilatation. The suggestion of warmth is quite logical since one of the effects of stress response is cooling of the skin because of constriction of blood vessels which is necessary to help diverting blood to the brain and muscles.

The third standard exercise focuses on normalizing the cardiac activity.

The forth standard exercise regulates the respiratory system.

The fifth standard exercise warms the abdominal area.

The last standard exercise reduces the flow of the blood to the head, thereby enhancing the feeling of relaxation.

Indications

It has been found to be effective in the treatment of disorders such as hyperventilation, asthma, ulcers, constipation, diarrhoea, high blood pressure, headache, cold extremities, general anxiety, irritability and fatigue. It can also help to control pain, increase your resistance to stress and reduce or eliminate sleep disorders.

It should be learnt under close supervision at a slow and comfortable pace. This method of relaxation involves imagination skills, which can easily be developed with regular practice.

Technique for Autogenic Training

You should maintain a very passive attitude, which means that you remain alert to your experience without analyzing it. Let whatever is happening happen. Each exercise introduces a verbal formula constantly to be kept in mind as you passively concentrate on one part of your body.

Position

Lie down with your head supported or sit on an armchair with a high back that can support your head or sit on a stool, slightly stooped over, with your arms resting on your thighs and your hands dropped between your knees.

Session I

Close your eyes and mentally repeat to yourself the following phrases. This session should be restricted to heaviness phrases as follows:
- My right arm is heavy
- My left arm is heavy
- Both my arms are heavy
- My right leg is heavy
- My left leg is heavy
- Both my legs are heavy
- My arms and legs are heavy

Note: If you have difficulty achieving a sensation of heaviness using the verbal formulas, you may want to add visual imagery. For example, imagine weights attached to your arms and legs and gently being pulled down. Think of the heaviness along the entire length of your limbs.

Session II

This session should be undertaken after you have been practicing session one for a few days. In this session we use the phrases based on the feeling of warmth as follows:
- My right arm is warm
- My left arm is warm
- Both arms are warm
- My right leg is warm
- My left leg is warm
- Both my legs are warm
- My arms and legs are warm

Practice heaviness phrases first followed by the warmth phrases. Again, use as many phrases as you feel comfortable with at first, gradually increasing them until you can use all the warmth phrases, before going on to session-III. If you repeat each of the session-I and session-II phrases three times with pause in between, it should take between seven to ten minutes to complete the exercise. Repeat the entire exercise three times a day.

Note: If you have trouble experiencing a feeling of warmth using the verbal formulas, try visual imagery. For example, imagine your right arm lying on a warm heating pad. Feel the warmth of the pad through your hand and arm. Imagine yourself in a nice warm shower. Envision yourself sitting in the sunshine.

Session III

This session is concerned with breathing. The phrase for this is 'My breathing is calm'. Repeat all the phrases of session-I and II, three times followed by the breathing phrase above. Continue practicing in this manner for a week or two before going on to session IV.

Session IV

This session uses a new phrase 'My forehead is cool and relaxed.

When people get upset , they often feel flushed in the face. This phrase evokes a feeling of a cool, damp flannel across the forehead.

Note: To enhance the feeling of coolness, imagine an ice cube placed in the centre of the forehead. Imagine the cool sensation, while repeating the phrase.

Autogenic training can be taken further than these basic formulas to include meditation or mental formulas such as

• My mind is calm and serene
• I am at peace

When you are at the end of an AT session, say to yourself, 'When I open my eyes, I will feel refreshed and alert.' Then slowly open your eyes, take a few deep breaths as you stretch and flex your arms, Keep sitting for a few minutes before going back to your regular activities.

An autogenics session should be for at least 20 to 25 minutes for significant benefits. It could even be longer. It could go up to 40 to 45 minutes.

Autogenic training can be a stepping stone towards greater self-mastery. It helps you to get a hold on yourself and to move on with renewed vigor.

MEDITATION

True stress management aims not only at managing a particular stress in a definite way but also on creating a state of mind that can help a person withstand and cope with stress. The aim of meditation practices is to induce the spontaneous state of meditation.

'Meditation' is a process that leads one to the inner fountain of the life and light. The state of mind once achieved, after practice brings about psycho-physiological changes and an altered state of consciousness.

Meditation—Rules for Practice

To experience meditation it is essential to follow a few basic rules and preparations.

Time

It is best to have fixed times for your daily meditation practices. The best time is early in the morning or in the evening before retiring to bed.

Practice before eating or a few hours after. It is best to eat moderately.

Duration

Fifteen minutes every day is better than one hour one day, half an hour next day and no time on the third day.

Position

Sitting in relaxed position, prescribe any meditational asana as in previous chapter, e.g. Padmasana, Sukhasana

Place of Practice

Clean and peaceful atmosphere. It should be well ventilated but not breezy, free from insects, warm but not hot, place a blanket or rug to sit.

Clothing

This depends on climate conditions. It should be light. It should not be tight or interfere in anyway with the breathing process.

Sleep

It is normal for most people to sleep when they relax. Probably the best way to prevent sleep during practice is to do asanas and pranayama before.

Awareness

Awareness means that you must be a witness to processes with the mind as well as the process of the meditational techniques. Sometimes the mind will be disturbed. It will incessantly jump from one thought to the next, or be totally obsessed by a problem. In this case, the best method to gain relaxation is to chant a mantra over and over again. Say like OM. If you do this with intensity, it has an almost incredible calming influence on the mind. It is so simple but very effective.

Technique

- Sit in any comfortable meditative asana
- Straighten the spine, sit erect
- Place your hand on the knees or in the lap
- Close your eyes and relax
- Be aware of your whole body
- Feel all the sensations of your body
- Be aware of any aches or pains
- Direct your awareness to the source of this discomfort and try to be aware of nothing else
- Let this pain be a focus for your awareness

- If your mind starts to wander, let it be but simultaneously try to maintain your awareness of the pain in your body
- Continue for few minutes
- Then direct your awareness to your right foot
- Be aware of nothing else but your right foot
- After a short time, transfer your awareness to the left foot
- Continue to be aware
- Transfer your awareness to your right leg and repeat the process
- Repeat the same procedure in turn with your left leg, with your whole back, abdomen, chest, right arm, left arm, neck, head and finally the whole body

This is one round. Intensify your awareness as much as possible.
- Do another round
- Be aware, suggest to yourself that 'I will not move my body'
- Your body must be like a statue
- After sometime you should find that your body becomes very stiff and rigid. You will find that you become detached from your body, weightless. The stiffening of the body is called psychic stiffening
- At this stage you are prepared for other meditational practices in which your focal point of awareness is internal

The level of relaxation and self-awakening depends on the amount of time given, the technique, regularity and duration of practice.

Benefits

Based on empirical evidence it has been found that those who practice some form of meditation have—
- A lower, more stable heart rate, a lower blood pressure
- Less chances of developing or relapse of heart diseases
- A slower, more stable respiratory rate
- Fewer psychosomatic symptoms
- Lower level of anxiety
- Better concentration at work
- Higher scores in self-actualization tests
- A better capacity for adjustment in society
- Better family and personal relationship
- Improved general health
- Greater enjoyment of life

YOGA

Yoga originated in India approximately 6000 years ago. Practitioners of yoga maintain that stress can be reduced by a mixture of mental and physical approaches. Stress management through yoga focuses on the techniques of breathing, Pranayama, Shavasana and yoga nidra. Breathing techniques help in diverting our mind from stressful situation.

All of the above mentioned techniques can be learned from previous chapters and can be practice as a part of your daily routine.

Apart from these techniques *visualization* or *imagery techniques* can be followed. Images are pictures formed within the mind.

Position

Sit erect, relaxed, close your eyes, and concentrate on a particular image. You may imagine being in a very peaceful environment such as garden. You can imagine any colors, shapes, smells and sounds, a very realistic picture can be quickly created in your mind with more practice. You can learn to project your own body image into this picture and ultimately to perform various tasks within the mind. For example, you visualize how you deal with a stressful situation. By creating various scenarios, you can learn to cope with all possible variations of a situation that may be stress-producing before confronting them in real life. The imagery can be continued as long as you wish.

Indications

It is found effective in stress-related and physical illnesses, including headaches, muscle spasm, chronic pain and general or situation-specific anxiety.

chapter eleven

Behavioural Techniques to Combat Stress

BIOFEEDBACK

Biofeedback is a common form of stress management and relaxation therapy. Biofeedback is the use of instrumentation to observe bodily processes, which are otherwise not visible or audible, and to help bring them under voluntary control. Information about the working of your body is fed to you by means of a visual or audio display so that you are actually able to observe–how your heart, muscular system, breathing, etc. behaves when you are stressed.

Biofeedback machines give immediate and ongoing information about biological activity, muscle tension, skin temperature, brain wave activity sweating (skin conductivity) blood pressure, heart rate and breathing (respiration).

Indications

Tension headache, migraine, hypertension, insomnia, muscle spasm, pain epilepsy, anxiety, phobia, asthma, stuttering and teeth grinding.

Method

The following are the standard modalities which are commonly used in biofeedback applications in the treatment of certain stress-related disorders.

Electromyogram (EMG) Training

The muscular tension present in the skeletal muscles of the voluntary nervous system is monitored by the EMG machine. These muscles include –

- **Frontalis muscles**—The muscle in your forehead that make you frown and tighten when you are worried or tense.
- **Mastoid**—Muscle that tightens your jaws and remains clenched when you are angry.
- **Trapezius**—Muscle that hunches your shoulders and tightens when you are alarmed or chronically anxious.

These muscles typically respond to stress and are accessible to monitoring. EMG training is done using two electrode placed at a convenient distance from each other and the third electrode placed on a neutral tissue (bone) to serve as an electrical reference point. The EMG feedback method is commonly used to treat anxiety, insomnia, asthma, hypertension, tension, ulcers, colitis and menstrual distress.

Thermograph (Temperature) Training

The thermograph monitors tiny fluctuations in body temperature. These are measured by recording finger, hand or foot temperatures. A sensor (heat sensitive electrode) is usually attached to the middle or little finger of the hand or foot. When you are tense the skin temperature goes down, due to a reduced blood flow because of constriction of the blood capillaries. It is believed that voluntarily raising skin temperature produces an anti-stress effect.

Temperature training has been successfully used in migraine, headaches, and circulatory problems associated with cold hands and feet.

Galvanic Skin Response Training (GSR)

Under severe stress the sweat glands in the body are activated leading to increased secretion. When a very tiny amount of current is passed through the skin, the increased sweat gland's activity registers an increased flow of current, which can be picked up by electrodes placed on the skin, usually on the forearm. This increased or decreased electrical skin conductance is picked up by the GSR machine to give appropriate feedback to you.

GSR training helps to gain control over your autonomic nervous system by monitoring the activity of your sweat glands. It has been successfully used in the treatment of anxiety and Phobia states.

Electroencephalogram (EEG) Training

The ongoing electrical activity of the brain is measured as brain waves. There are four states of brain activity typified by four types of electrical waves.
a. Alpha Waves (Associated with a state of calm relaxation)
b. Beta Waves (Wide awake and thinking)
c. Theta Waves (Light sleep or deep thought)
d. Delta Waves (Deep sleep or unconscious state)

The EEG biofeedback machine lets you know which of the four states you are in.

Alpha training is popular for teaching people how to relax. It is however, better used in conjunction with other biofeedback modalities.

Heart Rate Training

The heart rate monitor measures beats-per-minute and gives feedback on how relaxation affects the heart rate. A lowered heart rate is an indication of the relaxation response. Similarly there are machines that gives feedback about blood pressure. Biofeedback training provides no magical solution to the erasing of tension, but it requires time and patience as it involves two steps in relaxation. First, identifying when and where is the tension in your body and second, letting go of it. Biofeedback methods are best used along with the stress-reduction technique that works for you, it may be autogenic, progressive relaxation, visualization, yoga or meditation.

Apart from this "Thought Stopping" method has been practiced.

Thought Stopping, involves stopping a specific thought or thought chain. Initially it requires that you concentrate on the unwanted thought for a brief period of time and then suddenly stop and empty your mind. A verbal command, such as 'stop' or a loud noise is generally used to interrupt the unpleasant thoughts. Since thought stopping is based on the premise that negative thoughts affect how we react emotionally, by learning to control our thought we can drastically reduce overall stress level. Although appearing simplistic, this technique works very effectively.

chapter twelve

Lifestyle Management

NUTRITION

Your nutrition can determine how you look, act and feel.

Proper nutrition and adopting healthy eating habits can increase resistance to stress as well as directly reduce the chances of illness.

The Relationship between Stress and Eating Habits

People respond to stress in different ways: some smoke, some drink alcohol and some increases or decreases their food consumption. The net effect of overeating is weight gain. Weight gain is still another source of stress in our society.

Stressful situation—overeating

More stress—Weight gain

Overeating—More weight gain.

The most important thing to realize about this cycle is that the episode of overeating did not solve the problem unless the stressor was hunger.

Stress is often used as an excuse for not eating properly. I don't have time to eat. Instead of taking a break, consumes candy bars and potato chips.

What Makes-up a Healthy Diet

Although, individual requirements may vary significantly, the quality of a diet has to be kept in mind.

1. Eat a variety of foods. The greater the variety in your diet, the less the likelihood of a deficiency or an excess of any single nutrient.
2. Maintain ideal body weight. Being overweight puts stress on your body. Long-term weight maintenance depends on modifying your eating habits and on exercise.

   The following are some useful suggestions.
   - Eat slowly
   - Eat regularly
   - Do not eat, if you are feeling bored, instead engage in a pleasurable activity.
   - Do not eat, if you are angry. Communicate share your feelings.
   - When you are tired, go to bed, take a warm bath, drink water or lemon juice, rather than giving in to eating.
   - Eat smaller portions, keep serving dishes off the table.

- Eat when you are eating—do not read, watch TV, etc. So that you are aware of how much you are eating.
3. Avoid too much fats, saturated fat and cholesterol. Your diet should contain only about 30 percent of fat.
4. Eat foods with adequate starch and fiber.
5. Avoid sugar—It provides nothing nutritionally, but calories.
6. Avoid too much sodium/salt—Not more than 5 gm must be taken in a day. Limit your intake of salty foods, such as potato chips, salted nuts, pickle.
7. Avoid alcohol/cigarettes—Alcoholic beverages are high in calories and low in other nutrients.
8. Avoid Caffeine—Coffee, black tea, chocolate and colas are high in caffeine. Caffeine is a stimulant that chemically induces a 'fight' or 'flight' response in your body.
9. Take vitamin and mineral supplements—When under stress, you require more of all vitamins and minerals, especially vitamin B.
10. Vegetarianism—Vegetarianism has both a humanitarian and a hygienic basic. Meat contains fat in greater amount. Which is not healthy. Nutritious alternatives like seeds, grains, nuts, pulses, cereals and sprouts can be added.
11. Eat frequent, calm meals, small meals four or five time is better in a day than two or three large meals.

Sleep

Sleep is a healer. Adequate sleep is vital for health. It regenerates our body, clears emotional conflicts, help us think and then work at top efficiency and rejuvenates us.

Exercise

One very important benefit of exercise is muscle relaxation. In response to stress, our bodies often become tense. One way to relax after a tense day is to engage in exercise.

It helps to
- Reduce high blood pressure
- Increases physical strength and stamina
- Helps to regulates appetite and sleep
- Improves mental concentration
- Helps to relax and take off tension.

Time Management

It has been said that your time is your life. If you waste your time, you waste your life. Effective time management has been used in minimizing deadline anxiety, avoidance anxiety and job fatigue.

Strategies for Effective Time Management

- Plan and organize your time-table well in advance
- Plan in terms of time rather than tasks.
- Do not simultaneously start a number of demanding tasks.
- Complete one task at a time before going to the next.
- Allow space/gap between projects to recover physically and mentally.
- Group similar tasks.
- Allow time for the family and social commitments.
- Have some time just for yourself each day.

You must learn to utilize your time more efficiently to carry out things which are really important.

chapter thirteen

Putting It Altogether

1. Add Laughter in your life –
   a. Try to spend as much time as possible with cheerful people.
   b. Try not to take yourself too seriously always.

   Watch funny films, videos, read funny books.

   YOU WILL FIND DIFFICULT TO STAY SAD !!
2. Release your anger healthily—Anger is a normal human emotion. The biggest problem we face is—Learning how to discharge it in a manner that is both acceptable in society and healthy for ourselves.

   Here are a few steps to a healthy anger release—
   - Recognize the anger you are feeling. We often deny anger because we either feel too guilty about it or afraid of it, which is more dangerous.
   - Decide what makes you angry—Ask yourself, "Is this getting angry over".
   - Give the provoker the benefit of doubt, instead of inflaming your anger. Suggest to yourself that perhaps the other person has a bad day. Come up with a reasonable justification for the other's behavior.
   - Count to ten or practice some form of mental relaxation—calm down first, then discuss the conflict in a more rational peaceful way.
   - Listen—Listen carefully and understand
   - Learn the art of forgiving—Learn to forgive someone, many positive psychological and physiological changes take place. You feel warm and melty, your blood pressure and heart rate drop, you may even cry. But most important, we need to forgive for our own sake.

   So remember, the worst thing you could do with your anger is hit out. Accept it and handle it effectively and carefully.
3. Massage—Massage is a way of bringing touch back into your life and using it to soothe, calm and transmit caring. It is wordless communication of affection and understanding from one human to another. It releases tension from aching muscles, stimulates blood flow, eases stress, helps fluid drainage, generates sense of wholeness and peace. Massage, thus, greatly increases our sense of well being, both physical and mental.
4. Music—The power of music to promote change is not a new concept. The ways in which music affects us are varied. According to Diserens, it increases body metabolism, changes muscular activity, affects respiration, produces marked effect on pulse and blood pressure, reduces stress.

Therefore, appropriately selected music can enhance the relaxation experience through calming images and can also promote physical relaxation.

Getting Outside Help

Stress at times cannot be fought alone. You may find that in spite of using the various stress management, you are unable to cope with it. You may need others help. These others can be your own doctor, psychiatrist, psychologist or a trained counsellor.

Ultimately what needs to be realized is that when the going gets really tough, you should see for professional help or mobilizing social support in dealing with stressful times. Get on top of stress before it can get you.

SECTION 3
NATUROPATHY

chapter fourteen

Naturotherapy

Naturotherapy or Naturopathy or Nature care is a system of medicine, which aims at restoring health and eliminating disease by building up the vitality of the body. It's a constructive method of treatment, which aims at removing the basic cause of disease through the rational use of the elements, which is freely available in our nature.

The modern methods of nature cure originated in Germany in 1822, when Vincent Priessnitz established the first hydropathic establishment there. With his success in water cure, the idea of drugless healing spread throughout the world. Many medical practitioners from America subsequently enlarged and developed the various methods of natural healing in their own way. The whole knowledge was collected under one name—Naturopathy. Dr Benedict Lust is known as Father of Naturopathy.

Nature cure is based on the theory that man is born healthy and strong and that he can stay as such by living in accordance with the laws of nature. Sunshine, fresh air, exercise, proper diet, relaxation, constructive thinking and the right mental attitude, along with prayer and meditation all play their part in keeping a sound mind in a sound body.

Disease, on the other hand, is an abnormal condition of the body resulting from the violation of the natural law, where the cell metabolism of one or more organs has deviated from the normal path. This derangement of metabolism is commonly caused by.
- Dietary imbalance and deficiency.
- Poor living habits, such as shallow breathing, lack of exercise, rushed meals, negative thinking.
- Stress due to nervous tension, sudden environmental changes, occupational pressures.
  In naturopathic theory, all disease first appears at the cell level of the body. Typical stages of a disease process are –
- Mineral and vitamin concentration fall
- Enzyme action slows, vital enzymes cease to function
- Metabolism slows and alters
- Metabolic wastes build up
- The cell membrane degenerates
- Inflammation and pain are produced as warning
- Bacteria manifest and multiply, feeding off the waste
- Toxins produced by the bacteria cause further cellular injury
- Cell membranes disintegrate, the action of the organs is seriously impaired and their integrity is threatened.
- Degeneration of the organ sets in.
  The result of this disease process will show up in several ways.

Basic Principles

The whole philosophy and practice of nature cure is built on three basic principles.

- The first and most basic principle of nature cure is that all forms of disease are due to the same cause, the accumulation of waste materials and bodily refuse in the system. These waste materials in the healthy individual are removed from the system through the organs of elimination. Only way to cure disease is to employ method which will enable the system to throw off these toxic accumulations. All natural treatments are actually directed towards this end.

- The second basic principle of nature cure is that all acute diseases such as fever, cold, digestive disturbances, inflammations and skin eruptions are nothing more than self-initiated efforts on the part of the body to throw off the accumulated waste materials and that all chronic diseases such as heart disease, diabetes, kidney disorders are the result of continued suppression of the acute diseases through unhealthy methods such as medicines, vaccines narcotics and gland extracts.

- The third principle of nature cure is that body contains an elaborate healing mechanism which has the power to bring about a return to normal condition of health, provided right methods are employed to enable it to do so. The power to cure disease lies within the body itself.

chapter fifteen

Methods of Nature Cure

The nature cure system aims at the readjustment of the human system from abnormal to normal conditions and functions, and adopts methods to cure which are in conformity with the constructive principles of nature. First step towards curing disease is proper diet. To get rid of accumulated toxins and restore the equilibrium of the system, exclude acid-forming foods, including proteins starches and fats for a week or more and, take fresh fruits which will disinfect the stomach and alimentary canal. Do not overeat when you are sick, stick to very light diet of fresh fruit.

Another important factor in the cure of diseases by natural methods is to stimulate the vitality of the body. This can be achieved by using water in various ways and at varying temperature in the form of packs or baths. The application of cold water, especially to the abdomen, the seat of most diseases, and to the sexual organs, through a cold hip bath immediately lowers body heat and stimulate the nervous system. In the form of wet packs, hydrotherapy offers a simple natural method of abating fevers and reducing pain and inflammation, without any harmful side effects. Warm water application is relaxing.

Other natural methods, which are useful in curing diseases, are sun bath, massage, and manipulation exercise.

Thus, a well balanced diet sufficient physical exercise, fresh air, plenty of sunlight, pure drinking water scrupulous cleanliness, adequate rest and right mental attitude can ensure proper health and prevent disease.

DIET

Diet plays a vital role in the maintenance of good health and in the prevention and cure of disease.

The human body builds up and maintains healthy cells, tissues, glands and organs only with the help of various nutrients. The body can not perform any of its function, metabolic, hormonal, mental, physical or chemical without specific nutrients.

Nutrition, which depends on food, is the most important factor to cure disease. There is an elaborate healing mechanism within the body but it can perform its function only if it is abundantly supplied with all the essential nutritional factors.

It is believed that at least 45 chemical components and elements are needed by human cells. Each of these 45 substances, called essential nutrients, must be present in adequate diets. The list of these nutrients, include oxygen and water. The other 43 essential nutrients are classified into five main groups, namely carbohydrates, fats, proteins, minerals and vitamins. All 45 nutrients are vitally important and they work together. Therefore, the absence of any of them will result in disease and eventually in death.

A well-balanced and correct diet is the most important thing for the maintenance of good health and the healing of disease. Diet which should be a combination of all the essential nutrients.

It has been found that a diet which contains liberal quantities of—(i) seeds, nuts and grains (ii) vegetables and (iii) fruits would provide adequate amount of all the essential nutrients.

i) Seeds, nuts and grains—These are the most important and the most potent of all foods and contain all the important and the most potent of all foods and contain all the important nutrients needed for human growth. Millet, wheat, oats, brown rice, beans and peas are all highly valuable in building good health. Wheat, mung, beans, alfalfa seeds and soya-beans make excellent sprouts. Sunflower seeds, pumpkin seeds, almonds, peanuts and soyabeans contains complete proteins of high biological value. Seeds, nuts and grains are also excellent natural sources of essential unsaturated fatty acids necessary for health. They are also good sources of lecithin and most of the B vitamins, vitaminC. Which is the most important vitamin for the presentation of health. They are rich sources of minerals and supply bulk to the diet.

ii) Vegetables—They are very rich source of minerals, enzymes and vitamins. Most of the vegetables are consumed in their natural raw state in the form of salad. There are different kind of vegetables. They may be edible in the form of roots. Stems, leaves, fruits and seeds. Fleshy root contains high energy value and they are good source of vitamin B. Seeds are high source of carbohydrates and proteins and yellow ones are rich in vitamin A. Leaves stems and fruits are excellent sources of minerals, vitamins, water and roughage.

iii) Fruit—Like vegetables, fruits are an excellent source of minerals, vitamins, and enzymes. They are easily digested and bulk to food which gives good cleaning effect to blood and digestive tract. They contain high alkaline properties, a high percentage of water and a low percentage of proteins and fats. Apart from seasonal fresh fruits, dry fruits, such as raisins, and figs are also beneficial. Fruits should be eaten in their raw or ripen form.

The three basic health building foods mentioned above should be supplemented with certain foods such as milk, vegetables, oil and honey. Milk is an excellent food, which contains almost all nutrient. The best way to take milk is in its soured form that is yogurt and cottage cheese.

High quality unrefined vegetable oils should be added to the diet. They are rich in unsaturated fatty acids, vitamin C and E and lecithin.

Honey helps in calcium retention in the system, prevents nutritional anemia besides being beneficial in kidney and liver disorders, cold, poor circulation and complexion problems.

A diet of three basic food groups, supplemented with the special food mentioned above, will give a complete and adequate supply of all the vital nutrients needed for health, vitality and prevention of diseases. It is not necessary to include animal protein like egg, fish or meat in this basic diet as animal protein, especially meat, always has a detrimental effect on the healing processes. A high animal protein is harmful to health.

FASTING

Fasting refers to complete abstinence from food for a short or long period for a specific purpose. This a very powerful cleansing technique but should be used with care. A fast can extend anywhere from one day to about six weeks.

The common cause of all diseases is the accumulation of waste and poisonous matter in the body which results from overeating. The onset of disease is merely the process of ridding the system of these impurities. Every disease can be healed by only one remedy—by doing the opposite of what causes it, that is by reducing the food intake or fasting.

By doing fasting, the organs of elimination such as kidneys, skin, bowels, lungs are given opportunity to remove or expel the waste product. Thus, fasting is the process of purification and an effective and quick method of cure.

Duration

The duration varies from patient to patient according to their age nature of disease. Long duration fast are not advisable as it can be dangerous without proper guidance. It is always advisable to take sort duration fast.

Fasting is highly beneficial in all stomach and intestinal disorders and in serious conditions of the kidneys and liver.

Method

The most powerful but also the most difficult, is the water fast. Next is juice fast and then so-called mono diet. Recent researches have shown that juice fasting is the best way to fast because during fasting the body burns up and excretes huge amounts of accumulated wastes. We can help this cleansing process by drinking alkaline juice instead of water while fasting. Elimination of uric acid and other inorganic acids will be accelerated. And sugar in juices will strengthen the heart. Juice fasting is, therefore, the best form of fasting.

The patient should get as much fresh air as possible and should consume luke warm water at least 6 to 8 glasses.

A lot of energy is spent during the fast for elimination. It is, therefore, advisable to take rest and mental relaxation during the fast.

If any discomfort felt, it is advisable to discontinue the fast and take fresh cooked vegetables containing adequate roughage such as spinach and beets until the body functioning returns to normal.

Very simple exercises can be done. A warm water or neutral bath may be taken during the fast.

Benefits

There are several benefits of fasting. During a long fast, the body feeds upon its reserve. Being deprived of needed nutrients, particularly protein and fats, it burns and digest its own tissues by the process of autolysis or self-digestion. The body will decompose and burn those cells and tissues, which are diseased, damaged aged or dead. The essential tissues and vital organs the nervous system and the brain are not damaged. During fasting, the building of new and healthy cells are speeded up by the amino acid released from the diseased cells. The capacity of eliminative organs increases.

Fasting gives a physiological rest to the digestive assimilative and protective organs. As a result the digestion of food and the utilisation of nutrients is greatly improved after fasting.

Breaking of Fast

The main rules for breaking the fast are—do not over eat, eat slowly and chew your food thoroughly. Start with light food. The right food after a fast is as important and decisive for proper results as the fast itself.

Therapeutic Baths

Water has been used as a valuable therapeutic agent. In modern times, the therapeutic value of water was popularized by Vincent Priessnitz, Louis Kuhne and other European water-cure pioneers.

Water exerts beneficial effects on the human system. It equalizes circulation, boosts muscular tone and aids digestion and nutrition. It also tones up the activity of respiratory glands and in the process eliminates the damages cells and toxic matter from the system.

The common water temperature chart is cold 10°C to 18°C, neutral 32°C to 36°C and hot 40°C to 45°C. Above 45°C water loses its therapeutic value and is destructive.

The main methods of water treatment which can be employed in the healing of various diseases is given below.

Enema

An enema involves the injection of fluid into the rectum, only luke warm water should be used for cleaning the bowels. The patient is made to lie on his left side extending his left leg and bending the right leg slightly. The enema nozzle lubricated with oil or vaseline, is inserted in the rectum. The container which contains luke warm water is then slowly raised and water is allowed to enter into the rectum. Generally one or two liters of water is injected. After 5 to 10 minutes water can be ejected along with the accumulated morbid material.

A warm water enema helps to clean the rectum, which improves peristalsis, relieves constipation.

A cold water enema is helpful in inflammatory conditions of the colon, especially in cases of dysentery, diarrhoea, ulcerative colitis, haemorrhoids and fever.

Cold Compress

This is a local application using a cloth which has been wrung out in cold water or ice water, which is generally applied to the head, neck, chest, abdomen and back. The cold compress is an effective means of controlling inflammatory conditions of the liver, spleen, stomach, kidneys, intestine, lungs, brain, pelvic organs. It is also beneficial in fever and heart disease. It soothes dermatitis and inflammations of external portions of the eye.

Heating Compress

This is a cold compress covered in such a way as to bring warmth. It contains 3 or 4 folds of linen cloth wrung in cold water, which is then covered completely with dry flamel or blanket to prevent the circulation of air and help accumulation of body heat. The duration of the application is determined by the extent and location of the surface involved, the nature and thickness of the covering and the water temperature. After removing the compress, the area should be rubbed with a wet cloth and then dried with a towel. It can be applied to the throat, chest, abdomen and joints. It helps to relieve sore throat, hoarseness, tonsillitis, and laryngitis. Abdominal compress helps to cure gastritis, hyperacidity, indigestion, constipation, diarrhoea and dysentery. The chest compress helps to relieve cold, bronchitis, pleurisy, fever, and cough. While the joint compress is helpful in inflamed joints, rheumatism, sprains.

Hip Baths

This is the most useful form of hydrotherapy. A special type of tub is used for treatment. The tub is filled with water in such a way that it covers the hip and reaches up to navel, when the patient sits in it. Hip bath is given in cold, hot, neutral or alternative temperatures.

Cold Hip Bath

The water temperature should be 10°C to 18°C. The duration of the bath is usually 10 minutes, but in specific conditions it may vary from one minute to 30 minutes. If the patient feels cold or is very weak, a hot foot immersion should be given with the cold hip bath. The leg, feet and upper part of the body should remain completely dry during and after the bath. The patient should do moderate exercise after the cold hip bath, to warm the body.

It helps to relives constipation, indigestion, obesity and helps the eliminative organs to function properly. It is also beneficial in treating irregular menstruation. Chronic uterine infections, pelvic inflammation, piles, hepatic congestion, chronic congestion of the prostate gland, seminal weakness sterility, impotency, diarrhoea, dysentery. It should not be given in acute inflammations, of the pelvic and abdominal organs, ovaries and in painful contractions of the bladder, rectum or vagina.

Hot Hip Bath

This bath is generally taken for 8 to 10 minutes at a water temperature of 40°C to 45°C. The bath should started at 40°C and temperature should be gradually increased to 45°C. No friction should be applied to abdomen. Before entering the tub, patient should drink cold water. A cold compress should be placed on the head. A hot hip bath helps to relieve painful menstruation, pain in the pelvic organs, painful urination, painful contractions or spasm of the bladder, sciatica, neuralgia of the ovaries and bladder. A cold shower bath should be taken immediately after the hot hip bath.

Neutral Hip Bath

The temperature of the water should be 32°C to 36°C. This bath is generally taken for 20 minutes to an hour. The neutral hip bath helps to relieve all acute and sub-acute inflammatory conditions such as acute catarrh of the bladder and urethra and subacute inflammations in the uterus, ovaries and tubes.

It also relives neuralgia of the fallopian tubes or testicles, painful spasm of the vagina and pruritus of the anus and Vulva.

Alternate Hip Bath

This is also known as revulsive hip bath. The temperature in the hot tub should be 40°C to 45°C and in the cold tub 10°C to 18°C. The patient should alternately sit in the hot tub for five minutes and then in the cold tub for three minutes. The duration of the bath is generally 10 to 20 minutes. The head and neck should be kept cold with cold compress. The treatment should end with a dash of cold water to the hips.

This helps to relieve chronic inflammatory conditions of the pelvic viscera such as salpingitis, ovaritis, various neuralgias of the genito-urinary organs, sciatica and lumbago.

Spinal Bath

This bath provides a soothing effect to the spinal column and therapy influences the Central Nervous System. The bath can be given in cold, neutral and hot temperature. The water level in the tub should be an inch and a half to 2 inch and the patient should lie in it for 3 to 10 minutes.

The cold spinal bath relieves irritation, fatigue, hypertension and excitement. It is beneficial in almost all nervous disorders such as fits, hysteria, mental disorders, loss of memory and tension. The neutral spinal bath is a soothing and sedative treatment ideal for insomnia and also relives tension of the vertebral column. Duration of this bath is 20 to 30 minutes. The hot spinal bath helps to stimulate the nerves, especially when they are in a depressed state. Relives vertebral pain in spondylitis and muscular backache. Helps to relieve sciatic pain and gastrointestinal disturbance.

Full Wet Sheet Pack

This is a procedure in which the whole body is wrapped in a wet sheet, which in turn is wrapped in a dry blanket for regulating evaporation. The head should be covered with a wet cloth so that the scalp remains cold. The feet should be kept warm during the entire treatment. The pack is given for ½ hour to 1 hour till the patient begins to perspire profusely. He may be given cold or hot water to drink.

The pack is useful in fever especially in typhoid and continued fever helps in insomnia, epilepsy and infantile convulsions.

Hot Foot Bath

In this, patient should keep his leg in bucket filled with hot water at a temperature of 40°C to 45°C. Before taking treatment, a glass of water should be taken and the body should be covered with a blanket so that heat or vapor does not escape from the footbath. Head should be given cold compress. Duration of the bath is generally from 5 to 20 minutes. Patient should take a cold shower immediately after the bath.

It helps to stimulate the involuntary muscles of the uterus, intestine, bladder, pelvic and abdominal organs. Also relieves pain from ankle, foot, headaches caused by cerebral congestion and colds. In women it helps to restore menstruation.

Cold Foot Bath

In this 3 to 40 inches water at a temperature of 7.2°C to 12.7°C should be placed in a small tub or bucket. Feet should be immersed in the water for one to five minutes. We should rub the feet during the bath. It can be done with an attendant or by the patient by rubbing one foot against the other.

It helps in cerebral congestion and uterine hemorrhage. It is also helpful in the treatment of sprains, strains and inflamed bones when taken for longer period.

It should not be taken in inflammatory conditions of the genito-urinary organs, liver and kidney.

Steam Bath

It is one of the most important time-tested Hydrotherapy treatments, which induces perspiration in a most natural way. The patient should wear minimal or no cloth, is made to sit on a stool inside a specially designed cabinet. Before entering the cabinet, the patient should drink one or two glasses of cold water and protect head with a cold towel.

Duration of the steam bath is generally 10 to 20 minutes or until.

Profuse perspiration takes place. A cold shower should be taken immediately after the bath. Very weak patients, pregnant women, cardiac patients and those suffering from high blood pressure should avoid this treatment. If the patient feels giddy or uneasy during the steam bath, he should be taken out from treatment chamber and given cold water to drink and the face should be washed with cold water.

This helps to eliminate morbid matter from the skin surface, increases circulation and tissue activity. Helps to relieve rheumatism gout, uric acid problems and obesity. Also helps to relieve neuralgia, chronic nephritis, infections, tetanus and migraine.

Immersion Baths

This is also known as full bath. It is administered in a bathtub, which should be properly fitted with hot, and cold water connections. The bath can be taken at cold, neutral hot, graduated and alternate temperature.

Cold Immersion Bath

This may be taken for 4 seconds to 20 minutes at a temperature ranging from 10°C to 23.8°C. Before entering the bath, cold water should be poured on the patient's head. Chest and neck and head should be wrapped with a cold moist towel. During the bath, the patient should vigorously rub their body. After the bath body should be dried and wrapped in a blanket.

This bath helps to cure fever, improves the skin texture when taken for 5 to 15 seconds after a prolonged hot bath.

It should not be given to very young children (< 5 years) or very old patient and should be avoided in case of acute inflammation of some internal organs such as gastritis, inflammatory conditions of uterus and ovaries.

Graduated Bath

The patient should enter the bath at a temperature of 31°C. The water temperature should be lowered gradually at the rate of 1°C per minute until it reaches 25°C. The bath should continue until the patient starts shivering. The graduated bath is intended to avoid nervous shock by sudden plunge into the cold water.

It effectively brings down the temperature except in malarial fever. Besides from this, it gives general tonic effect, increases vital resistance and energies the heart.

Neutral Immersion Bath

It can be given from 15 to 60 minutes at a temperature ranging from 26°C to 28°C. It can be given for long duration, without any ill—effects, as the water temperature is akin to the body temperature. This bath diminishes the pulse rate without modifying respiration.

It gives sedative effect. It activates skin and kidney. It also gives

Good result in case of organic diseases of the brain and spinal cord, including chronic inflammatory conditions such as meningitis, arthritis.

It should not be given in eczema and other skin diseases, where water aggravates the symptoms, or in case of extreme cardiac weakness.

Hot Immersion Bath

This Bath can be taken from 2 to 15 minutes at a temperature from 36°C to 40°C. This bath should be started at 37°C and the temperature is then gradually raised to the required level by adding hot water. Before entering the bath, the patient should drink cold water and also cold compress should be given throughout the treatment. This bath can be useful in dropsy where there is excessive loss of tone of the heart and blood. It helps to relieve capillary bronchitis and bronchial pneumonia in children.

Relives congestion of the lungs and activates the blood vessels of the skin snd muscles. Bath should be terminated as soon as the skin becomes red.

In pneumonia and suppressed menstruation, the bath should be given at 37.7°C to 40°C for about 30 to 45 minutes.

In chronic bronchitis a very hot bath taken for 5 to 7 minutes should be accompanied with rubbing and friction. This relieves congestion of the mucous membrane and provides immediate relief. After Bath, oil can be applied.

This is also beneficial in case of obesity, Rheumatic joint pain gives immediate relief where there is pain due to stone in the gall bladder and the kidney.

It should not be taken in case of brain or spinal cord, or in cases of cardiac weakness and cardiac hypertrophy.

Epsom Salt Bath

The immersion bathtub should be filled with about 135 liters of hot water at 40°C. 1 to ½ kg of Epsom salt should be dissolved in the water. The patient should drink a glass of cold water, cover the head with a cold towel and then lie down in the tub completely for 15 to 20 minutes. The best time to take this bath is before retiring to bed.

This is very beneficial in case of sciatica, lumbago, rheumatism, diabetes, neuritis, cold and kidney disorders and other uric acid and skin affections.

Precautions: Certain precautions should be taken while taking therapeutic baths. Full baths should be avoided within 3 to 4 hours after a meal and one hour before full meal. Clean and pure water must be used for baths and water once used should not be used again. While taking baths temperature and duration should be strictly observed to obtain the desired effect. A thermometer should always be used to measure the temperature of the bath. Women should not take any of this baths during menstruation.

Power of earth: Earth forces have remarkable effects upon the human body, especially during the night. It gives refreshing, invigorating and vitalizing effect on body.

According to Adolf just by sleeping on the ground, the entire body is aroused from its lethargy to a new manifestation of vital energy, so that it can effectively remove old morbid matter and masses of old faces from the intestine, and receive a sensation of new health new life and new unthought of vigour and strength.

MUD PACKS

The use of mudpacks has been found highly beneficial and effective in the treatment of chronic inflammation caused by internal diseases, bruises, sprains, boils and wounds.

The advantage of mud treatment is that it is able to retain moisture and coolness for longer periods than cold water packs or compresses. The cold moisture in the mud packs relaxes the pores of the skin, draws the blood into the surface, relieves inner congestion and pain and promotes heat radiation and elimination of morbid matter.

Mud packs have been found to be a valuable treatment of diseases relating to general weakness or nervous disorders. Mud pack gives beneficial effect for swellings, eye and ear troubles, gout, rheumatism, stomach disorders, kidney and liver malfunction, diphtheria, neuralgia, sexual disorders, headache, toothache, general aches and pains. The pack is applied for 10 to 30 minutes.

Mudpack is prepared with clay obtained from about 10 CMS. Below the surface of earth to prevent from any impurities such as composts or pebbles.

It is most effective in decreasing the external heat and breaking up the morbid matter.

Hot and cold mudpacks are useful in relieving chronic pains, intestinal cramps, and lumbago. Alternate application helps to relieve discomfort caused by flatulence and intestinal obstructions. Also helpful in amoebiasis, colitis, enteritis and other inflammatory conditions of bacterial origin.

MUD BATH

It is applied in the same way as packs, but in a larger scale on the entire body. In this mud is made into a smooth paste mixed with hot water. The paste is spread on a sheet, which is wrapped around the body. One or two blankets are wrapped over this. A mud bath should be followed with a cleansing warm water bath and a short cold shower.

It helps to tone skin by increasing the circulation and energising the skin tissues helps to improve complexion, clear spots, Patches which is caused by various skin disorders. It is found to be very beneficial in Psoriasis, leucoderma and leprosy, Rheumatic pain. The duration of the bath should be from 30 minutes to 1 hour.

Therapeutic Massage

The word is derived from the Greak word massier which means to knead. It involves the scientific manipulation of the soft tissues of the body.

Benefits

It tones up the nervous system, influence respiration and increases circulation, and helps to remove the waste material from the body. It boosts metabolic processes. It helps to break the adhesion.

Contact Material

Cottonseed oil is most commonly used for massaging; Olive oil is also used. Talcum powder can be used in case of excess sweating.

Soap and water can be used in case of scaly skin, where body part is under POP or Prolonged immobilization.

Various Movements

There are five fundamental manipulations in massage. They are—Effleurage, Friction Petrissage, Tapotement and Vibration.

1. *Effleurage*—It involves sliding with the hands from distal to proximal. It helps to drain the fluid increases blood circulation. Helpful in oedema.
2. *Friction*—This movement circular in nature are performed in different manner by tip of the thumb, pad of the thumb and with the help of the finger or the palm. It helps to loosen the joint, removal of waste deposited material, help to break the adhesion, reduces swelling.

3. *Petrissage*—This is the process of kneading, pressing and rolling of the tissues and is performed with one or two hands with thumb and fingers.
4. *Tapotment*—This involves hacking lapping, clapping and beating. Mainly performed by doing wrist movement.
5. *Vibration*—This is achieved by rapidly shaking the pressing movements by use of the hand or fingers on the body. Vibrating hand should move constantly. This is beneficial in neuritis and neuralgia after the inflammatory stage is over. Stimulates circulation, glandular activity and nervous plexuses.

All these manipulation can be used for various therapeutic uses for whole body.

POWER OF COLOURS

Chromotherapy is a method of treatment of diseases by colours. It is best used as a supportive therapy along with other therapies. Such as diet, exercises, yoga and so on. According to practitioners of chromotherapy, the cause of any disease can be traced to the lack of a particular colour in the human system. Colour therapy is a technique of restoring imbalance by means of applying coloured light to the body.

Every substance on earth contains colour. Even the ray's cast on earth by celestial bodies contains colour in the form of white light. The rays of the sun contain seven different colours, violet, indigo, blue green yellow, orange and red. These are natural colours, which are highly beneficial in maintenance of good health and for healing diseases.

The Physiologic Effects of Colours

Red

The Pituitary gland activates. Further it activates adrenal gland and adrenaline is released. The following reaction begins immediately

- The blood pressure elevates.
- Blood flow increases, increases pulse rate.
- Breathing rate increases.
- Taste buds become more sensitive.
- The appetite improves
- The sense of smell heightens.

Orange

- The appestat elevates and appetite increases.
- Relaxation is induced and the potential for sleeps increases.
- Rate of Blood flow slows down.
- A sense of placidness, calmness, and security develops when orange is combined with blue.

Yellow

The electrochemical transference from eye to brain called vision takes place the quickest in the presence of yellow.
- Yellow is the first colour a person distinguishes when he sees something.
- Yellow gets a quick though temporally response from a subject under stress.
- Yellow adds to stress by preparing a person for flight of fight.
- Yellow—Painted rooms cause children to cry more offen.

Blue

- It slows the pulse rate
- Deepen breathing
- Reduce perspiration
- Lower body temperature
- Lessen sweating
- Eliminate the flight or fight response
- Reduces appetite.

Green

- Blood histamine elevates. Which dilates the blood vessels and contraction of smooth muscles such as the lungs.
- Allergic reactions to foods are reduced.
- Sensitivity reactions to monosodium glutamate are lessened.
- Hypersensitivity to food additives is reduced.
- Distress from eczema, diarrhea, and gastrointestinal disorders is lessened in severity and length.
- Vision chemicals that improve acuteness of sight are produced.

Brown

- Dispel mental depression
- Promote the synthesis of serotonin
- Reduce irritability.
- Eliminate chronic fatigue.
- Stimulate the formation of prostaglandin E1.
- Increases tryptophan amino acid levels that influence sleep, migraine headache immunity and moods.

Methods of Treatment

There are two methods of treating diseases by Colour.

I. By the application of light through different coloured glasses.

II. By external or internal use of colour charged water.

In the first method sheds of glass 30 CMS x 36 CMS, of the required colours are needed. These are placed at the window or any other convenient place in such a way that the sun rays can pass through them and fall directly on the patient's body. Duration of treatment is usually 30 minutes.

In the second method coloured bottles are needed. These bottles should be cleaned and filled up to ¾ level with fresh well water or rainwater. The bottle should be corked and then placed in bright sunlight for 3 to 4 hours. After this exposure, the water is said to be acquire medicinal properties and this colour—charged water can be used both internally and external application. Wound and ulcer can be washed with this water or an adult can take 30 ml of colour—charged water as a single dose. The dose can be repeated as required.

HEALING COLOURS FOR CERTAIN DYSFUNCTION

Red

It stimulates the sensory nerves, activates blood circulation, and excites cerebro spinal fluid. Red rays produces heat that vitalizes and energizes the liver, the muscular system and left cerebral brain hemisphere.

Red decomposes body accumulated salt crystals.

Indication for Red Colour Therapy –

- Anemia
- Asthma
- Blood dyscrasias
- Bronchitis
- Constipation

- Paralysis
- Physical debilitation
- Pneumonia
- Tuberculosis

Contraindication

- Emotional disturbances
- Hypertension
- High temperature
- Florid complexion
- Inflammation
- Mental illness
- Neuritis

Yellow

Yellow activates the motor nerves. A disturbance in the supply of Yellow vibration to any post of the body can bring partial or full paralysis.

On gastrointestinal tract for short period acts as digestive aid, exposure for longer period it acts as a both catharsis and cathartic. It helps to eliminate parasites and worms. Stimulates bile flow.

Indication

- Any type of Arthritis
- Flatulence
- Liver disorders
- Hemiplegia/Any Paralysis
- Kidney problems.

- Constipation
- Diabetes
- Digestive problems
- Eczema

Contraindications

- Acute Inflammations
- Fever
- Neuralgia
- Over excitement.

- Heart Palpitations
- Delirium
- Diarrhea

Orange

Orange is a combination of red and yellow rays, and its heating power is greater than either red or yellow alone. It stimulates thyroid gland and depresses Parathyroid. It has antispasmodic effect on muscle cramps, aids calcium metabolism, increases pulse rate.

Indications

- Asthma
- Kidney ailments
- Menstrual difficulties
- Prolapsed uterus.
- Respiratory diseases
- Rheumatism

- Bronchitis
- Colds
- Epilepsy
- Gall Stone
- Hyperthyroidism
- Hypothyroidism.

Contraindications are not known.

Green

Both dark and Pastel—builds muscles, bones and other tissue cells. It is cooling soothing and calming both physically and mentally. Relives tension, lower blood pressure, diastase capillaries and produce a sense of warmth.

Indications

- Asthma
- Colic
- Hayfever
- Exhaustion
- Heart problem
- Hemorrhoids
- Insomnia
- Irritability
- Venereal diseases.

- Back problems
- Malaria
- Malignancy
- Nervous disorders
- Neuralgia
- Syphilis
- Typhoid fever
- Ulcers

Contraindications are not known.

Blue

Blue vibratory rays increase the metabolism, build vitality, and promote growth slow the heartbeat. Blue is the balancing and harmonizing colour that returns the blood stream to normal. It reduces nervous excitement. It relaxes the mind.

Blue is the colour of truth, devotion, calmness, sincerity and the higher mental facilities.

Indications

- Bowel irregularly
- Cataracts
- Chicken pox
- Cholera
- Constipation
- Diarrhea
- Dysentery
- Epilepsy
- Eye inflammation
- Gastrointestinal disorders
- Gonorrhea
- Headache
- Heart palpitation
- Hydrophobia
- Itching

- Burns
- Laryngitis
- Measles
- Menstrual problems
- Kidney diseases
- Shock
- Skin diseases
- Syphilis
- Tonsillitis
- Typhoid
- Ulcers
- Vomiting
- Whooping cough
- Insomnia
- Jaundice

Contraindications

- Cold
- Gout
- Chronic rheumatism

- Muscle impairment
- Paralysis
- Tachycardia

Indigo

Indigo is electric, cooling and astringent. Stimulates parathyroid, blood purifier and a hemostatic agent.

Indigo rays control the psychic currents of the subtle spiritual bodies. They also control the forehead chakra and influence vision, hearing and smell on the physical emotional.

Indications

- Appendicitis
- Asthma
- Bronchitis
- Cataracts
- Convulsion
- Deafness
- Dyspepsia
- Ear diseases
- Mental Illness
- Nasal diseases
- Nervous Ailments
- Nosebleed
- Obsession
- Pneumonia
- Respiratory diseases
- Hyperthyroidism

Contraindications are not known.

Violet

Violet stimulates the spleen, upper brain, and bones. Depresses, the lymphatic, heart muscle and motor nerves. It's calming in case of mental illness.

Indications

- Bladder Problems
- Bone-growth dysfunction
- Cerebrospinal meningitis
- Mental illness
- Nervous disorders
- Rheumatism
- Scalp diseases
- Concussion
- Cramps
- Kidney disease
- Sciatica
- Skin diseases
- Tumors

Contraindications are not known.

Ultraviolet

Ultraviolet has chemical and bactericidal properties that break down bacterial toxins. It accelerates the lymphatic and circulatory systems, antibody production and metabolism.

Indications

- Goiter
- Rickets
- Syphilis
- Ulcers

- Gonorrhea   - Wounds
- Respiratory diseases

Contraindications—Malignant melanoma and other skin cancers.

Diet

A correct and balanced diet is essential during the treatment of diseases through chromotherapy. The various colours contained in different food.

Red   Beat, Radish, Tomato, Watercress, Watermelon, and Red skin fruits.

Orange   Carrot, Orange, Apricot, Mango, Pappaya and all orange—skinned vegetables.

Violet   Egg Plant, Berries, black carrot, and Purple grapes.

Yellow   Lime and lemon, grapes, Pumpkin, Melon, Banana, Mango, Guava.

Purple   Foods having both blue and violet colour.

Green   Most of the green vegetables, Spinach, Plantain, Pea, green mango, gooseberry, Beans.

Blue   Blue plum, blue beans.

EXERCISE FOR HEALTH

Several methods of exercises have been developed. Walking, Swimming, Cycling, and many more.

Advantage

1. Regular exercise contributes in good health and fitness. It helps to increase Basal metabolic rate.
2. Regular progressive physical exercise can bring about the balance of autonomic or involuntary, nervous system the tone of the vague nerve is strengthened.
3. Improved capillary action helps to increase strength and endurance.
4. Reduces gas and intraintestinal accumulation.
5. Increase respiratory capacity
6. Improves tone and function of veins
7. Stimulates sweat glands
8. Persistent exercise leads to improve quality of blood improve hemoglobin levels. Relatively greater alkalinity, improves total protein content and a greater cell count.

Precautions

• Vigorous exercise of any kind should not be taken for an hour and a half after eating.
• Weak patient, old person, suffering from heart disease, tuberculosis and asthma should consult their doctor before starting any kind of exercise.

- If you feel tired dehydrated during exercise stop immediately.
- Always start with light and short exercise programme then gradually increase.

YOGA THERAPY

Yogic kriyas, asanas and pranayama constitute the physical basis of yoga. The practice of kriyas and asanas leads to increases circulation, energises and stimulates major endocrine gland. Yogic exercises promote inner health and harmony, and their regular practice helps, prevents and cure many common ailments.

"Yoga and Naturopathy are like two wheels of a cart."

Further information can be collected regarding 'Yoga Therapy' from previous chapters.

SLEEP FOR REST

Sleep is one of nature's greatest inventions and blessings of life. It is a periodic rest of the body, which is absolutely essential for its efficient functioning. It has been called "Most cheering restorative of tired bodies."

Sleep is the indispensable condition to the recuperation of energy. It repairs the wear and tear of body and mind incurred during walking hours. Sleep is, thus, a vital element in a total way of life. It is a basic need in man's mental as well as physical life.

Duration

Dr. Nathaniel Kleitman, Associate Professor of Physiology at the University of Chicago says there is no more normal duration of sleep than there is normal height and weight.

On the whole women sleep from 45 minutes to 1 hour more than man does. The amount of sleep required varies at different ages as follows –

Newborn—18 to 20 hours

Growing Children—10 to 12 hours

Adults—6 to 9 hours

Aged People—5 to 7 hours

Sleeping well is an art. It needs a perfect blend of healthy habits and control of mind. A clean body and mind, relaxed mood, physical exercises, and perfect dietary control are some of the basic sleep-inducing methods.

The sleeping place should be well ventilated, warm but not, free from noise and insects. Bed should be neither too hard nor too soft. Pillow should not be too hard or high. Avoid wearing tight cloth and avoid having heavy meals before bedtime.

GOOD NIGHT

HAVE SWEET DREAMS.

SECTION 4
MAGNETOTHERAPY

chapter sixteen

Introduction

Earth itself is a huge magnet and possesses a magnetic field. All bodies in this space have their own magnetic field. Thus, man is constantly surrounded by magnetic waves and is influenced by them.

Very natural health can be restored or maintained with the help of a controlled magnetic field emanating from artificial magnets.

This therapy is based upon the principle that every disease is the result of an imbalance or in-coordination between the various electromagnetic forces present inside the body. Magnet therapy strives to eliminate such in-coordination and restore the natural balance of forces. Almost every disease can be treated with magnet. This therapy has a firm scientific base. It has gained tremendous popularity and acceptance in countries like Japan, America, Russia and Germany. In our country, still more awareness is needed.

chapter seventeen

Magnetism

The most important forces of nature include gravity, Nuclear force, Radiation and electromagnetic force. Magnetism is a part of the electromagnetic force.

Let us consider hydrogen atom. Nucleus of the hydrogen atom consists of a proton which constantly spin, which is not, only rotates around its own axis but also revolves around the center This movement also contribute to the magnetic field of the hydrogen atom. Thus, an atom is the smallest magnet exist. All the substance in this universe is made up of atoms, so electromagnetic waves are omnipresent.

Earth—A Huge Natural Magnet

1. The earth's magnetism originates because of the spinning of the earth about its own axis. One more theory which is accepted.
2. The earth's magnetism originates because of the electricity generated by the charged ions present in the atmosphere, especially the ionosphere.

Beyond the ionosphere of the earth, there is vast area full of harmful radiation. This area or belt is known as Van Allen belt. The earth's magnetic field effectively prevents this harmful radiation form reaching the earth's surface. Thus, this magnetic field serves a protective purpose for all living beings.

Earth's magnetic field is measured only about 0.5 gauss, which is adequate to protect and sustain life.

- Very important to know that earth's magnetic north Pole is situated at its geographic South Pole and the magnetic South Pole is situated at its geographic North Pole.

The Effect of Earth's Magnetic Field on Human Body

Baron Von Richenbach has found in his experiments that sensitive persons find discomfort and become agitated if lie down with their head towards the South. On the other hand, they feel relaxed and fall asleep when they lie down with their heads towards the north. In short, when a person remains parallel to the earth's magnetic field, he can do any work with least difficulty.

Experiments have shown that when the head of a person lies towards the north, alpha, delta and theta waves dominate inside the brain gradually the thinking process slows down and person feel relaxed. Thus, the brain requires the cooling and peace-giving waves emanating at the geographic North Pole of the earth (i.e. it's magnetic South Pole). If lying down in the north-south direction can be kept under the pillow such that the cool South Pole lies upward i.e. faces the person's head.

chapter eighteen

How do Magnets Act

It is very important to know what changes occur in our body when magnets are applied to the body part.

Every cell and every organ of our body is a magnetic unit and has a specific vibratory frequency. When there is a perfect harmony between the vibratory frequencies of the various tissues and organs of the body. We are in good health. If this harmony is imbalance because of changes in the natural vibratory frequency of an organ or a part of the body causes disease.

Magnet therapy strikes at the root of the disease. It strives to restore the natural vibratory frequency of the various organs and to re-establish a balance in their electromagnetic forces.

The Direct Effects of Magnetism

When magnet are kept in contact with a part of the body, the cells and organs of that part regain their natural vibratory frequency.

The electromagnetic waves coming from the magnets are capable of very deep and extensive penetration and reach almost every cell of the concerned part of the body. The protoplasm of the cells gets polarised. Such polarisation imparts strength to the cells. When magnets are placed near the body, the regeneration proces in that part is stimulated. New, healthy ones replace old worn out cells. It helps to heat the wound faster.

Magnet also suppresses the activities of harmful bacteria, which causes disease.

The Indirect Effects of Magnetism

A magnet affects the physical and chemical properties of liquids. Centers of crystallisation increases, the density, the viscosity, the surface tension is suitable altered.

When electromagnetic waves enter the blood stream, they produce eddy current. These eddy currents warm up the blood and increase the number of ions in the blood.

These ion-rich polarised and warm blood circulates it provides good heath. It helps in the removal of metabolic waste product. Which helps to reduce muscular tension, fatigues and pain.

Cholesterol deposition on the inner surface of the blood vessels are eroded and dissolved. Thus, blood supply to organs are improved. This warm blood stimulates the endocrine glands to function properly.

It helps to bring down ESR and WBC count in infectious illness, where it goes up abnormally. In short, magnetised blood rejuvenates and invigorates each and every cell of the body, various systems of the body become more efficient, Resistance Power increases.

chapter nineteen

Magnetised water

Substances can be classified into three category:
  I Ferromagnetic
  II Paramagnetic
  III Diamagnetic
- Ferromagnetic substances are strongly attracted towards a magnet, e.g. Iron, Nickel, Cobalt.
- Paramagnetic substances are mildly attracted towards a magnet—such as water, oil.
- Diamagnetic substances move away from a magnet, Gold, Sliver, Zinc.

Effects of Magnetic Field on Water

It has been found that magnetic field increases the centers of crystallisation in fluids. When exposed to a strong magnetic field physical properties of water like density, viscosity, surface tension, electrical conductivity and chemical properties like pH, nitrogen ion concentration undergo changes. This water is termed as 'magnetised water'.

This magnetised water, when drunk, favorably affects the health.

This water is useful in most diseases especially in digestive, excretory and the nervous system. It helps to improve digestion, reduces gastric acidity, helps to cure constipation and it is also very helpful in treating menstrual problem. It taken regularly prevents deposition of cholestrol on the inner surface of blood vessels. Magnetised water is diuretic in nature, which is found very useful treating kidney troubles. It is also very useful treating kidney stones.

This water strengthens and invigorates the natural resistance power to the body. Hence, it is useful in case of viral disease, common cold, cough, asthma and most other diseases.

How to Magnetise Water

Strong magnets are used to magnetise water. Water should be in plastic bottle or glass bottle and should be kept in contact with strong magnet for about 24 hours.

Water influenced by both the Poles (south as well as north) simultaneously should be consumed. For this two magnets should be placed on either side of a bottle containing water such that the North Pole of one magnet faces the South Pole of the other magnet.

Water magnetised by only one Pole may be used for certain problem as in hyperacidity or gastric ulcer water magnetised by South Pole alone should be used. On the other hand, for sluggish digestion, water magnetised with North Pole alone can be used.

For magnetising water, the magnets are to be kept in contact with the water bottle from outside; they should not immersed into the water.

It should not be heated or kept in a refrigerator.

Once water is magnetise, effect remain for about 3 to 4 days.

Doses—The water should be taken 3 to 4 times a day, in doses of about 100 ml (Half a glass)

This water can be used to wash eyes, to clean wounds and burns and to flush the intestine (through Enema)

chapter twenty

Magnetised Oil

Oil too, can be magnetised and rendered more useful.

OIL INFLUENCED WITH BOTH THE POLES

Take a glass bottle filled with required oil. Keep strong magnets in contact with this bottle such that North Pole of one magnet faces the South Pole of the other magnet. Retain such contact for 15 to 20 days.

This oil can be used for hair, baby massage or for instilling in the nose and ears.

OIL INFLUENCED WITH NORTH POLE

In this method only the North Pole of the magnet should be in contact with the bottle containing oil. The magnet should preferably be positioned such that it faces the north direction.

This oil is recommended as a massage medium in general weakness, paralysis, and baldness.

OIL INFLUENCED WITH SOUTH POLE

In this method, only the South Pole of the strong magnet should be in contact with oil bottle. The magnet should be positioned to face the south direction.

This oil is recommended in case of massaging joint disorders, pain, and skin problem and insomnia (scalp massage).

Milk magnetised for a few minutes with the north Pole, if drunk at night, enhances sexual ability.

chapter twenty-one

Principles of Applying Magnets for Treatment

There are two important methods of applying magnets.

1. The unipolar method, where only one Pole (either the south or the north) is used at a time
2. The bipolar method, where both the Poles are used simultaneously.

First we should know the properties of both Poles.

Properties of South Pole

- i. It is inhibitory and suppressive
- ii. It imparts coolness and peace
- iii. If kept in water for sometime, it makes the water slightly alkaline. It decreases the acidity of fluids.
- iv. It produces contraction and shrinkage of body tissue.
- v. It slows down the circulation in small blood vessels and capillaries.
- vi. It inhibits the activity of bacteria, controls infection and decreases inflammation
- vii. It arrests growth of boils, carbuncles and tumors.
- viii. Decreases pain and body temperature.

Thus, the South Pole is useful in infectious and inflammatory conditions. It is commonly used in skin condition arthritis, infectious diseases, tumors, anxiety, convulsions, pain neuralgia insomnia and many more.

Properties of the North Pole

- i. The North Pole possesses stimulatory or augmentative properties.
- ii. It imparts warmth and energy.
- iii. If placed in water for sometime, it increases acidity of fluid.
- iv. It produces expansion of body tissue.
- v. Speeds up the circulation in small blood vessels and capillaries.
- vi. It encourages the activity and growth of bacteria, worsens infections and increases swelling.
- vii. Stimulates the growth of boils and tumors.
- viii. No effect on pain, sometime it increases pain and it increases body-temperature.

The energy, strength and warmth giving properties of the North Pole can be utilised to treat paralysis, hernia, leucoderma, boldness, muscle weakness, general weakness unconsciousness and many more diseases.

Since the north and the South Pole have opposing properties, correctly recognising the poles is very important before treating any diseases.

Treating with 'Unipoles' treatment it is necessary to correctly diagnose the disease. This is very important because an incorrect diagnosis may lead to an use of the incorrect pole of the magnet, resulting into a failure to cure the disease or ameliorate the symptoms.

However, bipolar method should be employed whenever there are clear indications for doing so. For example, if the part of the body to be treated is painful as well as weak or stiff, both the poles can be used. But there should not be any active infection.

The north and the south poles can also be used one after the other, during a single treatment session. In injury, spinal pain, low back pain, treatment with the South Pole for the first 10-20 minutes and with the North Pole for the next 10-20 minutes may be given.

Some physicians treat each and every disease by keeping the magnet in contact with the patient's palms and the soles.

It is must to consider the changes that occur in the body, when the magnets are applied in above mention way.

1. When the north pole is kept in contact with the right palm (or sole) and the south pole is kept in contact with the left palm (or sole) cool forces inside the body gradually increase and dominate all the process inside the body slow down.

2. When the north pole is kept in contact with the left Palm (or sole) and the south pole is kept in contact with the right palm (or sole) hot forces gradually increases in the body all the processes in side the body are paced up.

In conditions like fever, excessive, perspiration. Allergy, high blood pressure Rheumatoid, we can go for first type if magnet placement, which cool down the body.

In conditions like frostbite, paralysis, varicose vein, obesity, diabetes we can go for second type of magnet placement which stimulates the hot forces in the body.

Position of the Patient

Sitting or lie down as per patient's convenience and the need of the treatment. Iron bed or chair should be avoided, wooden bed or chair should be used. If the magnets are to be applied to the soles, they should be kept on a wooden plank and not on the floor.

During the treatment, the magnets should preferably be positioned such that the North Pole faces the north direction and the South Pole faces the south direction. In this position, the field of the magnets is parallel to that of the earth and gives better result.

Choice of Magnets

The shape, the size and the power of the magnet selected for treatment depend upon the need.

1. Delicate and sensitive, small organs, brain and heart should not be treated with strong magnets a small round or rectangular magnet with a central hole can be used for treating such organs.

2. Superficial diseases do not need very strong magnet(such as skin problem) but if the disease is deep-seated strong magnet may have to be used.

3. Strong magnet may be required for old and chronic disease.

Duration

In the initial stages a 15- minute treatment session, once a day is adequat. For infants 5-10 minutes should be enough.

For chronic diseases, joint-disorders, paralysis and other such serious diseases, the duration should be 30-40 minutes. In such conditions the treatment can be given two or three time a day. The duration of a single treatment depends upon the kind of disease and the condition of the patient.

Time

If strong magnets are to be used stomach should be empty. It is best to take treatment early in the morning or early evening.

There is no serious side effect of magnetic treatment, so it can be taken any time of the day.

chapter twenty-two

Advantage of Magnetotherapy

The antibiotics and other medicines are found to give major side effects. Many time body opposes these medicines on the other hand magnetotherapy is an external mode of treatment which doesn't play with the various chemicals and enzymes present inside the body and it is also safe and harmless. Side effects are unknown with magnetotherapy .

It's not a slow or long-term treatment. Results can be seen immediate. Magnetotherapy is very simple. It can be employed for patients of any sex or age. No preparation is essential before starting the treatment.

It needs very little care in the form of cleaning or sterilization. If treating skin disease, little care should be taken. After treating skin diseases magnet need to be cleaned.

There is no need to go to clinic; it can be taken at home. There is no particular time for treatment. It can be taken any time of the day.

Once purchased, the magnet can be used for years, because they retain their power for a long time.

Magnetic treatment is not addictive. No harm arises up abruptly.

Magnets can be used to disperse fatigue and irritation.

All together magnets can prolong life and prevent senility.

PRESERVATION OF MAGNET

1. Magnet should not be allowed to clash with each other or to fall, otherwise steel magnet may loose their power and ceramic magnets may break.
2. Magnet should preferably be kept in a wooden case or a wooden cupboard, when not in use.
3. Steel magnets should not be allowed to get wet to prevent them from resting. Similarly, the part of the body to which the magnet is to be applied should be completely wiped, free of sweat.

SECTION 5

ACUPUNCTURE

chapter twenty-three

History of Acupuncture

Acupuncture is the ancient Chinese art of healing and is probably more than 5,000 years old. It is believed that once a Chinese soldier's leg was wounded by an arrow, on removal of the arrow, suddenly he got relieved from shoulder pain, which he was suffering from many years, he could move freely his shoulder again without any pain.

This incident forced physicians to think, was there a relationship between the arrow wound and the relief from pain, over a period of time they found that there are many points located near the nerve ending, which when stimulated, has therapeutic effects. They have used different medium to stimulate these points with sharpened fish bones; bamboo sticks and stone needles (known as BIAN). They have got very good results. They were surprised to know that there is some kind of link or channels in the human body, which carries these healing effects. Thus began the art and science of acupuncture.

Huang Di Nei Jing Su Wen popularly called the yellow emperor's classic of internal medicine, is the foundation stone of traditional chinese medicine. It is said to be the oldest medical text in the world. This book is written in two parts, first known as Su Wen or simple question, contains the principles of medicine, in second part acupuncture is described know as Ling Shu or magic gate. This deals with the prevention and cure of illness.

The acupuncture points were first systematically described during the Tsin Dynasty (265-420A.D.) and about 349 basic acupuncture points and about 649 in whole body were listed.

The ancient philosophic theory of the five element and the concept of Yin and Yang has been used since 770-467 BC of chinese history. The theory of meridians and Luo connection and flow of 'Qi' through them is the base of acupuncture.

The whole world is divided into five elements—wood, fire, earth, metal and water. Which transform into one another and this process maintains the existence.

Moxibustion is originated in northern China. They discovered that applying heat relieves symptom of abdominal pain, distension and fullness.

Based on these observations hot pressing and moxibustion method were developed. Even now we use this method for treating illness and pain.

Leading institutes of Australia, USA, Japan, France, Korea, Germany, Hong Kong and China are engaged in further acupuncture research.

Only future would be able to tell us, up to what heights this method of curing human disease will rise.

chapter twenty-four

What is Acupuncture?

In Latin ACUS means needle and *Punctura* or *Pungue* means pricking. Acupuncture is an ancient chinese art of healing, where various diseases of the body cured by inserting very fine needles in the specific points of the body. There are more than 1,000 acupunture points in the human body located along 12 main pathways or channels in each half of the body and two channels in the mid-line of the body. These points when stimulated either by needles or warming cure the disease. This needle stimulation can be done manually or electrically. Burning a herb "Artemisia vulgaris" can do the heating and this technique is known as moxibustion. These two techniques can be practised separately or in combination.

THE CONCEPT OF CHI (QI) OR LIFE ENERGY

According to Chinese philosophy, every thing in the universe comprises energy. This energy in the Chinese language is called *Qi* or *Chi* (pronounced chee).

In the Indian philosophy it is known as *Prana*.

The principle of Prana is quite similar to the "Qi" or the energy of life.

The primary function of "Qi" can be seen in all movements, whether involuntary –such as heartbeats and respiration or voluntary –such as walking, eating. "Qi" is universal and present at all the time in different form. It is the invisible force responsible for all the movement of life. It permeates all living cells and circulates in the body and a constant process of the transformation of air, food and water into the "Qi" takes place throughout one life. "Qi" or "Chi" has two components *Yin* and *Yang*.

YIN AND *YANG* (Fig. 24.1)

"In every organism, a part is the whole and the whole is the part- Dwait theory of Hinduism.

Yin and *Yang* they are dynamically opposite yet harmonising energies. This harmony brings about a balanced state of the universe. Good health is the state of energy balance and bad health imbalance between both energies. They act as opposite poles negative and positive and are complementary to each other. *Yang* signifies for male, light, active, warm, dry sun, heaven, up, strength, and all that is positive.

Ying signifies for female, passive, dark, cold, moist, moon, earth, dirty, peace, harmony, endurance, weakness and all that is negative.

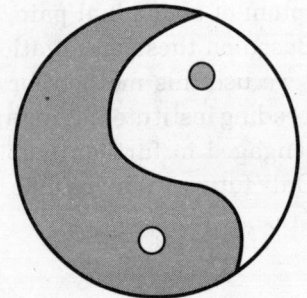

Figure 24.1: Yin and Yung

A closed circle divided into two equal halves by a sinus curve represents it. Two different colours are used for both circles. In each half circle, there is a small circle of opposite colour this opposite colour shows that *Yin* in suppressed while *Yang* is on its peak and *Yang* is suppressed while *Yin* is on its peak.

'JING LUO' AND 'ZANG-FU' ORGANS

The meridians (channels or pathway) are passages in the body where the vital energy *'CHI'* or 'Qi' flows. In Chinese they are known as *'JING LUO'* (Jing-path Luo-connection).

Meridian goes vertically from below upwards or above downwards are the main meridian and termed as *'Jing'*.

Other than this there are 12 paired main meridians and extra ordinary meridians. The collateral that link the main meridians together are called *'Luo'*.

These 12 paired meridians Originate from the internal viscera of the body. The viscera are divided into two categories.
1. 'Zang' or solid organs.
2. 'Fu' or hollow organs.

Table 24.1

Main	Paired	Arm	Yin Yang
			Lung (L)
			Large Intestine (Li)
			Pericardium (P)
			Small intestine (Si)
			Heart (H)
			Triple warmer (Tw)
		Leg	Leen (Sp)
			Stomach (St)
			Gallbladder (Gb)
			Liver (Liv)
			Urinarybladder (Ub)
			Kidney (K)
	Unpaired		Conceptional Vessel (Cv)
			Ren Mai (Ren)
			Governing Vessel (Gv)
			Belt Vessel Dai Mai
			Vital Vessel Chong Mai
Extraordinary	Paired		Yang Ankle Vessel Yang Chiao Mai
			Yin Chiao Mai
			Yin Ankle Vessel Yang Wei Mai
			Yang Regulating Vessel Yin Wei Mai
			Yin Regulating Vessel

Zang organs such as heart, lung, spleen, liver stores the 'Qi' energy, while 'Fu' organs such as stomach, intestine, bladder discharge it.

Zang organs are *YIN* (negative) and those originated from 'FU' organs are *YANG* (positive) in polarity. These *YIN* and *YANG* meridians are linked (LUO) by collateral.

To converse the polarity of *Yang* and *Yin* each organ contains a part of both the principles in variable proportions.

For the good health of the body and mind, there must be sufficient and equal energy in each of these meridians.

FIVE ELEMENT THEORY

According to Indian Philosophy, everything in this Universe belongs to any of the five elements- Fire, Air, Water, Earth and Sky. This is the theory of 'Panchmahabhoot'

Similarly, according to the traditional Chinese Philosophy, the whole Universe is divided into five elements namely Wood, Fire, Earth, Metal and Water.

In the living body they symbolise the internal organ and their cycles explain the phenomenon of nature.

The Table 24.2 will make this symbolism more clear.

Table 24.2

	Wood	*Fire*	*Earth*	*Metel*	*Water*
Yin organ	Gallbladder	Small intestine, Tripal warmer	Stomach	Large intestine	Urinary bladder
Yang organ	Liver	Heart, Pericardium	Spleen	Lung	Kidney
Sence organ	Eye	Tongue	Mouth	Nose	Ear
Taste	Sour	Bitter	Sweet	Acid	Salty
Emotion	Anger	Joy	Obsession	Sadness	Fear
Searetion	Tears	Sweat	Saliva	Mucus	Urine
Body Tissue	Muscle	Blood	Fat	Skin	Bones
Colour	Green	Red	Yellow	White	Black
Direction	East	South	Centre	West	North
Season	Spring	Early summer	Late summer	Autumn	Winter

The Chinese believe that all these five elements are related in the destructive cycle called 'KO' as well as the generative cycle 'Sheng' (Fig. 24.2).

These five elements are constantly transformed into one another and as shown above there are two cycles of events generative and destructive.

A. *In destructive (Ko) cycle*
- Fire destroys metal by heating and melting
- Metal destroys wood by cutting
- Wood destroys earth in the form of plant root breaking soil.

Earth destroys water by stopping its natural flow in the form of a dam.

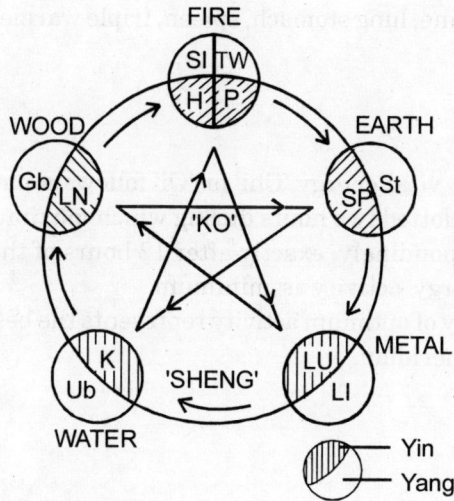

Figure 24.2: Five element theory

B. *In constructive (Sheng) cycle*
- Fire is fueled by wood.
- Wood is burnt to yield earth (ashes)
- From the earth metal can be mined
- Metal when heated turns to liquid like water.
- Water nourishes growth of plants i.e. wood.

MOTHER AND SON LAW

'Qi' or 'Chi' always flow from mother to the son. For proper flow mother should be healthy, properly well nourished and the child should be strong and healthy enough to receive. In the flow of energy the son becomes the mother of the following meridian after receiving the energy and in turn the recipient organ again becomes the mother of the next following organ.

Thus,

Liver is the mother of heart
Heart is the mother of spleen
Spleen is the mother of lung
Kidney is the mother of liver
Lungs the mother of kidney

HUSBAND AND WIFE LAW

Husband dominates the wife. *Yang* dominates *Yin* and left wrist pulse dominates right wrist pulse. Organs related to the husband are heart, gallbladder, liver, small intestine, urinary bladder, and kidney and large intestine, lung stomach, spleen, triple warmer and pericardium are related to wife.

ORGAN CLOCK

The Chinese observed that vital energy 'Chi' or 'Qi' follows a particular time sequence. Each organ meridian has been allotted two hours during which maximum energy flows through that particular meridian correspondingly, exactly after 12 hours of this high tide, a low tide occurs in the meridian when energy activity is minimum

This two-hour periodicity of optimum activity represents the best time for taking acupuncture action on the concerned meridian.

chapter twenty-five

Positive Effects of Acupuncture

The effects observed on needling on the body are both subjective and objective.

Subjective Effects

1. *Pain*—at the site of needling is the first sensation felt by patient. This particular sense in Chinese is called "deqi".
2. *Numbness*—when the needle is passed into the body, patient feels numbness along the meridian.
3. *Heaviness*—Sometimes the needling point is becoming heavy mainly in extremities.
4. *Soreness*—Sometimes patient complains of soreness.
5. *Distension*—Patient feels something is moving from the needling point to the end of the meridian.

"Deqi" with combination of other senses indicates that the needle have been placed accurately for the success of treatment.

Objective Effects

These are physiological effects:

Analgesia

Acupuncture needling raises pain threshold through,

A. Sensations arising out of this needling compete with the painful stimuli, reach the spinal cord first and block the incoming painful sensation according to Gate control theory which says all pain impulses are first controlled and modulated in the substantia gelationosa (first functional gate) of the spinal cord, before they travel up through spino-thalamic tracts(second functional gate). When these impulses reaches cerebral cortex, patient feels pain. Para ventricular and the contra lateral nuclei of the thalamus and the medial reticular foramen of the midbrain also work as functional gate. By needling the acupuncture point, the over-crowding of the impulses occurs at the functional gates and needling the acupuncture point blocks them proceeding further. This causes increase in pain threshold and gives analgesic effects.
B. By needling certain chemicals and neurotransmitters such as endorphins and enkephalins are secreted in the body, which bind themselves with specific receptors in the brain to block the painful sensations.

This Analgesic property is made use in treatment of arthritis, headache toothache, back pain, sprains, etc.

Sedation

Acupuncture for some people give drowsy effect. It can be use in treatment of insomnia, mental disorders, anxiety, hysteria, addictions, epilepsy, and behavior problems.

Homeostatic

Adjustment of the internal environment of the body towards normal balance. Vital functions like respiration, heart rate, blood pressure, metabolic rate, sweating, body temperature. It can be normalise with the help of acupuncture. It can also stop pathological degeneration process, especially in arthritis and spondylosis.

Immunity Improvement

By needling certain acupuncture points, increases in healthy white blood cell, antibodies, gamma globulins is seen, thereby, helps to increase body resistance to disease. So, it can be used in treatment of mild to moderate infections. It has been found very useful in controlling and minimizing bleeding during surgery and bringing down post-operative complications.

Psychological Effects

It has been found that during the treatment patient feels less tensed and worried, and more cheerful and communicative.

Motor Recovery

Acupuncture has shown fast motor recovery or stimulates non-responding muscles to improve function. It is found very useful in paralysis.

Internal Acceptance and Support

WHO, issued a provisional list of 41 diseases amenable to acupuncture treatment. These include respiratory ailments, pain and chronic pain condition. Premenstrual syndrome and other gynecological disorders, gastrointestinal disorders and many other health problems, respiratory tract disorders. Acute sinusitis, common cold, tonsillitis, broncopulmonary disorders—acute bronchitis, bronchial asthma; eye-disorders—acute conjunctivitis, myopia, optic nerve atrophy mount cavity disorders—toothache, gingivitis, pharyngitis, gastro intestinal disorders—spasm of esophagus, gastritis, hyperacidity, gynecological disorders—cervicitis, leucorrhea, painful periods, neurological and orthopedic disorders—headache, trigeminal neuralgia, facial palsy, peripheral neuropathy, backache, arthritis, post-polio paralysis, tennis elbow, sciatica.

chapter twenty-six

t-Sun: A Unit of Measurement

Unit of the measuring acupuncture points on the body is t-sun or cun, one t-sun or cun is the distance between the palmer creases over the proximal and distal inter phalangeal joint of the middle finger of the patient. The combined breadth of the index and middle finger is 1.5 t-sun. The combined breadth of the four fingers together is 3 t-sun or 3 cuns.

    One fen is equal to 0.1 t-sun

    Eight t-sun equal to 1 Fu.

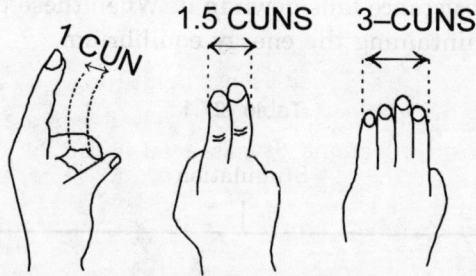

Figure 26.1: Cun measurement

chapter twenty-seven

Methods of Stimulation in Acupuncture

According to the traditional Chinese concept, the acupuncture points are located on the body following the meridian system. When these points are stimulated by different methods, they result in bringing the equilibrium in the disturbed energy, i.e. "QI". According to the modern concept, the acupuncture points are low electrical resistance spots all over the body. During any disease the electrical resistance falls down in it. When these points are stimulated, they can cure the disease by maintaining the energy equilibrium.

Table 27.1

Stimulation

Ancient   Modern

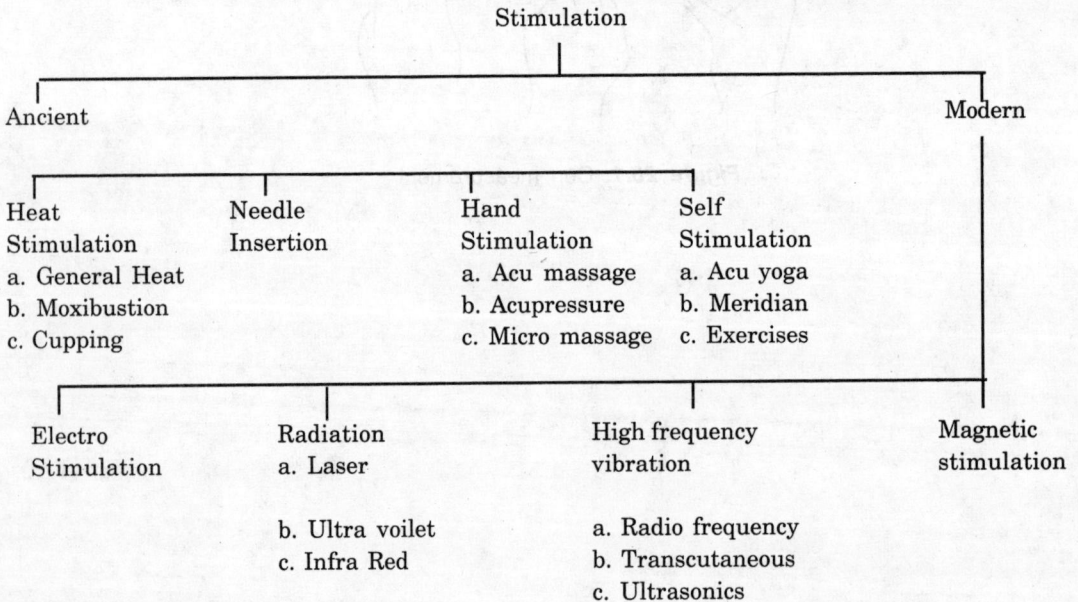

Heat Stimulation	Needle Insertion	Hand Stimulation	Self Stimulation
a. General Heat		a. Acu massage	a. Acu yoga
b. Moxibustion		b. Acupressure	b. Meridian
c. Cupping		c. Micro massage	c. Exercises

Electro Stimulation	Radiation	High frequency vibration	Magnetic stimulation
	a. Laser		
	b. Ultra voilet	a. Radio frequency	
	c. Infra Red	b. Transcutaneous	
		c. Ultrasonics	

Heat Stimulation

a. *General or Direct heat*—In this type of Stimulation, a hot coin or scarring the acupuncture point with red hot iron was done.
b. *Moxibustion*—In this therapy part was treated by heating a point by burning moxa wool to produce heat.

c. *Cupping*—It was known as the 'horn method'. It means treatment through local congestion or blood stasis by using a small jar or cup in which vacuum is created by burning a piece of cotton soaked with alcohol kept inside the jar so that oxygen inside is consumed and the vaccum is created. In modern time the cup is attached by suction to the skin surface over the selected point.

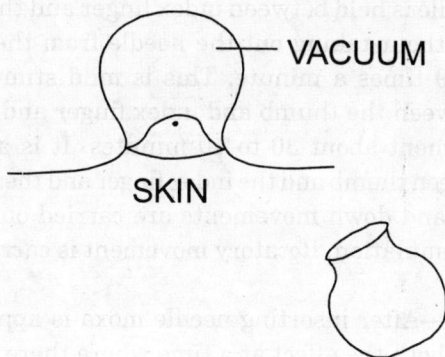

Figure 27.1: Cupping

Needle Insertion

This is of two type

a. Tonification (bu) or by inforcing energy
b. Dispersion (xie) or by reducing energy.

There are different type of needle insertion.

a. *Superficial Needling*—It is about ½ cun or only subcutaneous needling in the body tonifies the energy. It can be used in paralysis cases.
b. *Deep Needling*—Deep insertion of a needle reduces the energy. It can be used in acute cases in painful condition.
c. *Along the direction of energy flow*—Each meridian's energy flows in particular direction. If we insert a needle along the direction of flow of energy, it increases the energy.
d. Against the direction of energy flow—If the needle is inserted against the energy flow it reduces the energy.
e. If needle is inserted during inspiration it increases the energy and during expiration it reduces energy.
f. If needle is inserted rapidly and removed slowly, it increases energy and inserting it slowly and removing fast will decrease energy.

Type of Needle Hand Stimulation

a. *Tapping*—In mild stimulation very slow tapping can be done about 20-30 times in a minute on the head of the inserted needle with fingertip.

b. *Rotating*—Needle is held between the thumb and the index finger and rotated by the fingers either clock-wise or anti-clockwise about 15 to 20 times a minute.

c. *Flicking*—This is a strong stimulation where needle is held between the thumb and the index finger and up and down movement is carried out with needle moving in the range of 2 cm and at a very fast rate about 50 to 60 times per minute.

d. *Up and down movement*—Needle is held between index finger and thumb slow up and down movements are carried out without taking out the needle from the body at that point in the range of 1 cm and 5 to 20 times a minute. This is mild stimulation.

e. *Vibration*—Needle is held between the thumb and index finger and vibration is given side ways and up and down movement about 30 to 40 minutes. It is a strong stimulation.

f. *Snapping*—Needle is held between thumb and the index finger and then with very fast rotatory movements by the fingers up and down movements are carried out about 40 to 60 times a minute. It is a very strong stimulation. Rotatory movement is carried out simultaneously with up and down movement.

g. *Heat stimulation to the needle*—After inserting needle moxa is applied to the head of the needle and ignited. This gives both the effect at a time where there is increase or decrease of energy is desired.

Hand Stimulation (Fig. 27.2)

a. *Acupressure*—Slight pressure at the point results in increase energy and hard pressure at point decreases the energy.

b. *Acumassage*—Massaging at the point we can either increase or decrease the energy. This is of different type –

   i. Tui—Massaging with palm and fingers

   ii. Na—Massaging with the heel of palm

   iii. Ning—Pinching the body points in the hand and giving massage.

   Tui helps to increase energy flow while Na reduces energy. With Ning, it helps to reduce pain very fast.

c. *Micro Massage*—Flexion of elbow where biceps is tightly contracted. It produces few small vibrations in the fingers. While these small vibrations, slow massage is given. With light micro massage we can notify the energy and with deep micro massage reduction in energy is found.

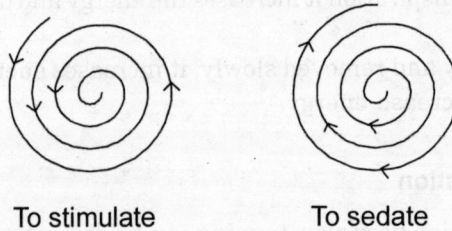

To stimulate   To sedate

Figure 27.2

d. *Self Stimulation* –
  i. Acu yoga—Different type of yogic positions the pressure is located at the particular points is known as Acu-yoga
  ii. Meridian exercise—These exercises resemble yogic positions with slight difference.

MODERN METHODS OF STIMULATION

Electrostimulation

It was invented in 1966 in china to give electrical stimulation to needles with different types of stimulation like –
a. Adjustable impulses
b. Dense and disperse impulses
c. Discontinuous impulses
d. Ripple impulses
e. Saw tooth impulses

Both low frequency electrical stimulation which is used for rehabilitation and electro acupuncture treatment are employed using the method of playing two terminal (Plate and needle terminal) on the body. Electricity flows between these two terminals.

The power of the electric stimulation is proportional to the density of the current, the

Figure 27.3: Wave patterns in electrostimulation

part of the body around the smaller terminal that gives a high electric density receives more electric stimulation. The smaller plate terminal which transmits a higher electric density and stronger stimulation is called the 'treatment terminal' or 'negative terminal'.

Negative electricity gives better stimulation using less electricity, therefore the affected part should be treated by the treatment terminal (Negative Terminal).

The advantage of electro stimulation over the hand stimulation. It has the stimulating capacity around the acupuncture point within 5 mm around the point in all directions.

- Dense and disperse impulses—10-25 c/m
  Uses—chronic pain, inflammation and analgesics
- Ripple impulses 10-25 c/m
  Uses—analgesics, acute pain, spasticities
- Discontinuous impulses 10-25 c/m
  Uses—intermittent stimulation for muscle atrophies. Chronic nerve problems, sciatica, paralysis.
- Saw tooth impulses 10-25 c/m
  Uses—same as 3 above.
- Adjustable frequency impulse (2-50 c/m)
  Uses—routine therapy—anaesthesia.

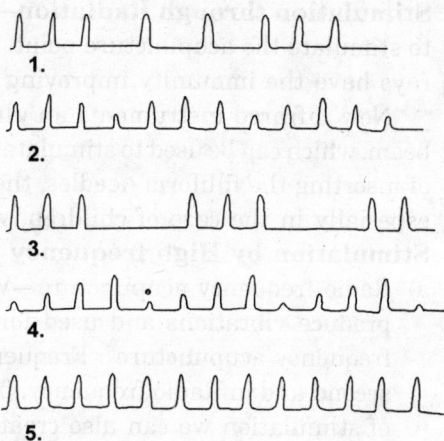

1. **Magnetic stimulation**—Magnet can stimulate energy in meridian. For Tonification of a point south pole of one magnet should be kept over diseased point and the north pole seeing the direction of energy flow in that meridian proximal to it. So to tonify we have to stimulate along the direction of energy from the north pole to the south pole. For immunity improvement use the north pole on the diseased place.

2. For the upper half of the body use the north pole at the left palm and south pole at the right palm, for lower half of the body, north pole at left sole, south pole at right sole.

3. **Stimulation through Radiation**—Simple infrared lamp or ultraviolet lamp can be used to stimulate the acupuncture point. Infrared light is used for reliving pain and ultraviolet rays have the immunity improving and tonification effects.

   New infrared instruments an ultraviolet instruments use to radiate rays in a narrow beam, which can be used to stimulate the acupuncture points to get the desired effect. Instead of inserting the filliform needles, these rays can be used safely without needling the body, especially in the case of children, very old or very sensitive patient.

4. **Stimulation by High frequency vibration** –

   a) Radio frequency acupuncture—When the radio frequency sound wave is converted to produce vibrations and used for the acupuncture point stimulation called as "Radio frequency acupuncture". Frequency of electro acupuncture is about 1 to 1000 HZ per second and in Radio frequency, from 1000 HZ to 10,000 HZ per second. In these ranges of stimulation we can also create acupuncture anesthesia.

   b) Transcutaneous acupuncture—They are skin electrodes, applied over the acupuncture point. It can also be used in conjunction with electrical stimulation in acupuncture therapy. This method consists of a small metal plate affixed to the particular acupuncture point and stimulated electrically similar to conventional Electro acupuncture using trans-cutaneous acupuncture needle.

   The advantage is skin puncture is not done so, there is relief from needling pain and any type of infection. But in certain cases such as paralysis, routine acupuncture shows far better results. Transcutaneous stimulation can be given for very old, very small or sensitive patients.

   Ultrasound and Radio frequency stimulator also transmit transcutaneous stimulation. The bipolar biphasic electrical impulse by the stimulator created when transmitted through the nerves gives the desired effect. An accurate knowledge of the dermotomes is must for giving transcutaneous stimulation with acupuncture points.

5. **Ultrasound stimulation**—The term sonopuncture or ultrasonic stimulation is used for acupuncture, carried out by using a narrow, cylindrical, high frequency beam of sound instead of needle. The human ear is capable of hearing sound waves between 20-20,000 cycles per second. Sound waves with a frequency of 20, 000 cycles per second or more are two high pitched to be heard by the human ears are called ultrasound.

   Sound waves applied to the acupuncture meridian system have been found to be safe and effective. This method has an advantage over needle acupuncture in that it is totally painless.

For sonopuncture, specially constructed high quality sound heads are used that generate a narrow cylindrical beam of ultrasound. These special- purpose sound heads emit intense vertical beams ranging around 2-5 mm in width. Each of these special purpose sound heads is handcrafted to exacting standards to ensure that the beam is uniform.

Sonopuncture is a quick method of therapy that requires 30-60 seconds of stimulation at each acupuncture point. It has an effective depth of penetration of 6-8cm. While doing sonopuncture a conducting medium like a gel or oil is used.

This deep penetration is possible, because ultrasound waves are conducted through fat without absorption and are absorbed by the underlying muscle. This makes sonopuncture an effective alternative to acupuncture even in very fat patients.

Indication

Treatment of Infections, Varicose veins, Spinal problems, Promote healing of fractured bone, Asthma, Bronchial Problems.

chapter twenty-eight

Methods of Acupuncture

In ancient India Rishi's used fish bones and pointed bamboo sticks for effective treatment. In ancient China needles made out of bamboo, animal horns, and a variety of metals were used. Later silver and gold needles were used. Nowadays the most commonly used needles are made up of stainless steel with handle of silver which is quite effective and economical.

There are several shapes and sizes of needle.

Filliform Needle

This is the most common needle used, available in different length ranging from 0.5 t-sun to 8.0 t-sun. They are used according to site and desired depth of insertion.

It is available in different diameters thick needles produces more pain and it is used for stronger stimulation. Thin needles are less painful. Thickness varies from 26 to 32 gauge.

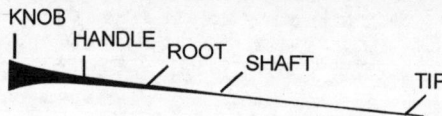

Figure 28.1: Parts of needle

Parts of needle

Filliform needles with double spiral handle are used for scalp acupuncture. They are 1.5 to 2 t-sun in length and 28-30 gauge thick.

Same for upper extremely 1 to 2 t-sun in length and about 30 mm is used. Longer needles are used for areas like buttock, where muscle mass is thick. 3 to 5 t-sun in length and 20-30 mm is used.

Gauge—standard unit for measuring thickness of Metal.

Press (Intra-dermal Needles) (Fig. 28.2)

They are small button—shaped needles with a point projecting from center. The length of tip is about 1 mm. In chronic stubborn diseases like bronchial asthma and certain type of addiction continuous stimulation is required on ear points.

The needle should be fixed on the ear point with adhesive plaster and it can be kept for 3 to 5 days and patient is advised to massage over it 3 to 4 times a day.

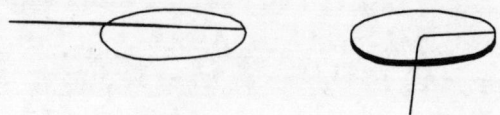

Figure 28.2: Round body press needle

Triangular Needle (Sanlingchen)

This is also known as prismatic needle. A thick, sharp-edged triangular needle. These needles are used for bleeding from jing-well point. The needle is held between the thumb and the index finger and a superficial rotation is made until bleeding occurs. After few drop of blood comes out from the point, the spot is pressed to stop any further bleeding. These are mainly used for certain type of inflammatory conditions, acute diseases and allergic skin condition.

Cosmetic Needles

Thin, comma shaped needle for cosmetic problems like pimples, wrinkles, freckles are used.

Plum

Blossom or seven—Star needle (Fig. 28.3)

Seven small needles protruding out from a hammer. This is used to tap along the meridians or on specific areas of the skin until the area becomes red. All skin diseases like eczema, psoriasis, dermatitis, alopacia, etc.

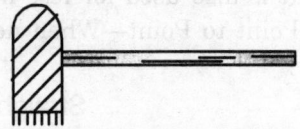

Figure 28.3: Seven star dermal needle

Hidden Subdermal

Needles—Small needles 0.3 to 0.5 t-sun in length. They should be kept for 3 to 5 days on acupuncture point with sticking plaster.

This is found very helpful treating asthma, headache, hepatitis, myopia, etc.

Hot-needle

Thick 18-gauge needle to treat conditions like ganglion, cystic goiter. It is heated over a lighter or spirit lamp and suddenly poked in the part and then bandaged.

Sterilization of Needles

The needle are kept in 70% alcohol for 24 hours or it can be sterilized in an autoclave due to danger of contamination with the hepatitis and AIDS.

Boiling of needles are avoided as it may destroy the sharpness of the tip of the needle.

Traditional Acupuncture Techniques

The practice of acupuncture with needles is an ancient technique. Needle should be between the thumb and index finger. Bring the tip of needle near the acupuncture point and use it rapidly for piercing the skin. From then onwards the way in which the needle is passed depends upon the type of treatment desired. After inserting the needle it should be manipulated by hand 'Te-chi' or 'de-qi' is achieved.

Te-chi or de-qi—When the tip of the needle is inserted to the correct depth a sensation of pain, sourness, numbness, heaviness, fullness and distension may be experienced by the patient. Frequently de-qi is felt as a radiating sensation and experienced along the acupuncture meridian. There should be no pain if the procedure is done properly except for certain points on the hand, foot, face and ear points.

Direction of the Needle (Fig. 28.4)

a. Straight or Perpendicular—It is used for extremities at 90 degree
b. Slanting or oblique—30-60 degree
   It is used where there is less muscles are present as chest and head
c. Horizontal—10-20 degree
   It is also used for less muscular area
d. Point to Point—When needle from one point penetrates through another point

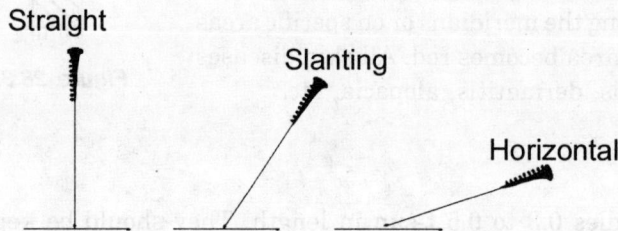

Straight

Slanting

Horizontal

Figure 28.4: Showing direction of needle insertion

Type of Stimulation

a. Up and own movement within 1 cm
b. Rotation to and fro rotation of needle between thumb and index finger
c. Flicking—Produced by thumb and index finger, usually 20 flicks per period of stimulation
d. Vibration—1 to 2 mm rapid up and down movement done with the first for 1 to 2 minutes
e. Snapping—Snapping of the middle finger on the needle gently

Manipulation of Needle

Manipulation of needle is essential for increasing or suppressing effect on energy. If the treatment is for local pain or stagnation (blockage of energy flow) it will be necessary to manipulate the needles. Manipulation can be of following ways.

Thrusting Technique

In this technique the needle is thrust up and down by a push-pull force exerted on the handle. The correct depth is first obtained through de-qi and the needle then lifted just a few millimeters and immediately returned to the original depth. The amplitude of the movement is increased for very strong stimulation. But needle is not withdrawn from the body.

Twirling Technique

In this technique needle is inserted to the correct depth and then rotated almost 180 degrees. This is repeated for about half a minute, allow the needle to return to neutral more or less by itself. If the needle is rotated clockwise gives stimulating effect and if anticlock wise it causes sedation

Figure 28.5: Thrusting technique

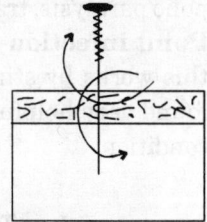

Combination Technique

This is the most difficult technique to perform but gives better result. While needling when the patient is breathing out and raising or lifting during inspiration a greater degree of stimulation (tonifying) is obtained and needling during the inspiratory phase and withdrawing it during expiration, a greater degree of sedation is found. Manual manipulation has to be done fairly rapidly and has to be sustained for the duration of the entire treatment.

Figure 28.6: Twirling technique

Degree of Stimulation

a. **Strong stimulation**—Up and down snapping, flicking for acute cases and younger patients.
b. **Medium stimulation**—Up and down, snapping, flicking similarly as above, but gently or slowly applied.
c. **Weak stimulation**—Slow rotation, slow flicking used for old patient and in chronic cases. It is also used for sedation and insomnia.

Duration of Stimulation

a. Short—After patient get Te-chi, then all types of stimulation techniques are given for about 20 seconds and then remove the needle. It is found useful in case of general problems such as toothache, headache, etc.
b. Intermediate—After getting Te-chi rotate needles for several seconds, stop for 2-3 minutes, then repeat the rotation. It can be given for 10-20 minutes according to the response desired. Used in chronic cases such as Sciatica, Migraine, arthritis, etc.
c. Continuous—Following Te-chi continuous twisting of needle for 1 to 2 hours is done until patient has relief from his symptoms. This is used for renal colic, acute headache, etc.

Non-traditional Acupuncture Techniques

- **Aqua puncture**—In this form of acupuncture a small volume of fluid—usually a Vitamin solution or distilled water—is injected into the site of the acupuncture point. The rationale is to stimulate microcirculation in that area, which in turn, promotes healing.

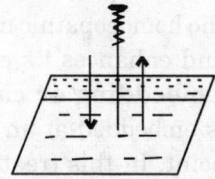

- **Homoeopuncture**—Homoeopuncture is a new technique where needles are dipped into the homoeopathic medicine and inserted at a specific acupuncture point. It acts immediately and enhances its effect.
- **Embedding or catgut therapy**—This is a technique in which a surgical catgut suture is embedded at an acupuncture point with the aim of giving constant stimulation to the point. In this treatment a needle with catgut is inserted at a specific acupuncture point. The needle is then withdrawn leaving the catgut embedded in the skin. This catgut is left for 3 to 4 week till it dissolves. During this time the catgut is embedded, it gives constant stimulation to the acupuncture point and helps in achieving quicker results. This therapy is found very useful in resistant cases of chronic bronchial asthma, chronic backache, post polio paralysis, traumatic paraplegia, cerebrovascular accidents, and chronic hyperacidity.
- **Point infection therapy**—In this therapy drugs are injected at the acupuncture points, this works by stimulating the micro-circulation and increasing the body resistance. It is found very helpful in case of asthma, lumbago, allergies, skin disorders and other painful condition.

Micro-acupuncture Techniques

In the olden days people were bon earring to improve their vision. Incidentally this point corresponds to the 'eye' point of acupuncture. Diagnosis and treatment of the disease by means of ear or auricle is termed as "Auriculo Therapy". This form of treatment has been widely practiced in different parts of the world.

AURICULOTHERAPY

Advantages

a. Almost all the diseases can be treated by this technique.
b. It can be given with combination of all forms of acupuncture.
c. It gives quick relief.
d. Economical for patient, easy to learn.
e. It can be used for both prevention and treatment of the disease.
f. Needles can be safely left in points for many days to obtain desired result.

Indication

a. Prevention and treatment of disease
b. Diagnosis and differential diagnosis
c. Acupuncture anesthesia

Contraindication

Patient may get infection of the ear if not treated properly.

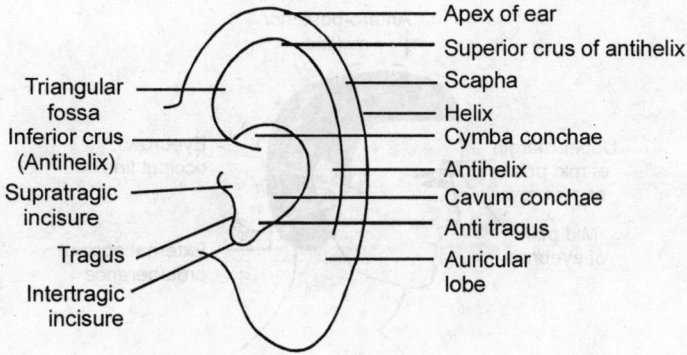

Figure 28.7: Surface marking of external ear

DISTRIBUTION AND DESCRIPTION OF ACUPUNCTURE POINTS

Auricular Lobe (Figs 28.8a and b)

It corresponds to the face and has nine areas shown in Figure 28.9.

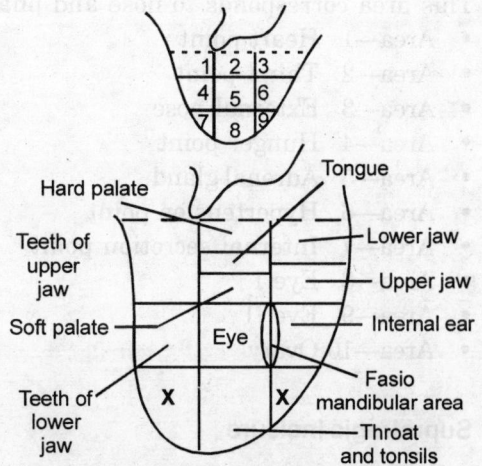

Figures 28.8a and b: Points on the auricular lobule

- Area—1 Postero inferior part of this area represents the teeth of the upper jaw. It is the analgesic point for toothache and anaesthetic point for tooth extraction.
- Area—2 The upper 1/3 of this area represents the hard palate. Central one third represents tongue and lower 1/3 represents sift palate.
- Area—3 The upper ½ of this area represents lower jaw and lower ½ represents upper jaw.
- Area—4 The central point is analgesic point for toothache and anaesthestic point for extraction of the teeth of the lower jaw.
- Area—5 Central point of this area represents eye.
- Area—6 Central point of this area represents internal ear.
- Area—7 It has no acupuncture point.
- Area—8 Central point of this area represents tonsils and throat.
- Area—9 It has no acupuncture point.

Facio-mandibular area—It is located between area 5 and area 6. It is used in the treatment of trigeminal neuralgia and facial paralysis.

Cheek area—It is located at the junction of 5th and 6th area.

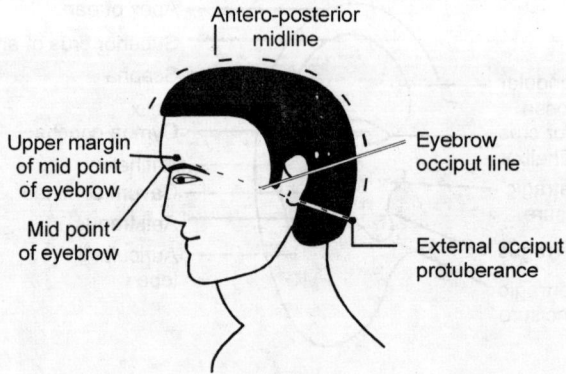

Figure 28.9: Stimulation area of scalp-needle standard lines

Tragus (Fig. 28.10)

This area corresponds to nose and pharynx

- Area—1 Heart point
- Area—2 Thirst point
- Area—3 External nose
- Area—4 Hunger point
- Area—5 Adrenal gland
- Area—6 Hypertension point
- Area—7 Internal secretion point
- Area—8 Eye I
- Area—9 Eye II
- Area—10 Ovary

Supratragic Incisure

This area represents heart and external ear.

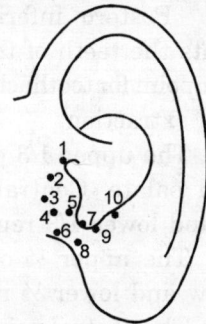

Figure 28.10: Points on tragus, intertragic and supratragic incisurre

Anti-tragus

This area represents head region.

Anti-helix—This area represents trunk (Fig. 28.11)

- Area–11   Toes
- Area–12 Ankle
- Area–13 Knee
- Area–14 Hip
- Area–15 Lumbago Pain
- Area–16 Buttock area
- Area–17 Gluteal Region

- Area–18   Lumbar Vertebra
- Area–19   Thoracic Vertebra
- Area–20   Neck
- Area–21   Cervical Vertebra
- Area–22   Brain
- Area–23   Ding chuan (soothing asthma point)

Triangular fossa (Deltoid fossa) (Fig. 28.12)

- Area—24   Blood Pressure lowering point
- Area—25   Hepatitis point
- Area –26   Shenmen
- Area –27   Hip Joint
- Area –28   Hot Point
- Area—29   Buttock
- Area—30   Sciatic Nerve
- Area—31   Sympathy
- Area –32   Uterus
- Area –33   Asthma
- Area –34   External genitalia
- Area—35   Urethra
- Area—36   Urinary bladder
- Area—37   Kidney
- Area—38   Ascites Spot
- Area—39   Pancreas
- Area—40   Lower segment of Rectum
- Area—41   Large Intestine
- Area—42   Appendix
- Area—43   Duodenum
- Area—44   Mouth
- Area—45   Oesophagus
- Area—46   Stomach
- Area—47   Gall bladder
- Area—48   Liver
- Area—49   Spleen
- Area—50   Heart
- Area—51   Lung
- Area—52   Subcortex
- Area—53   Internal Secretion
- Area—54   Adrenal
- Area—55   External nose.

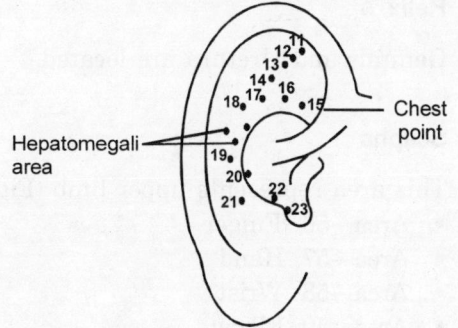

Figure 28.11: Points on anti-tragus and anti-helix

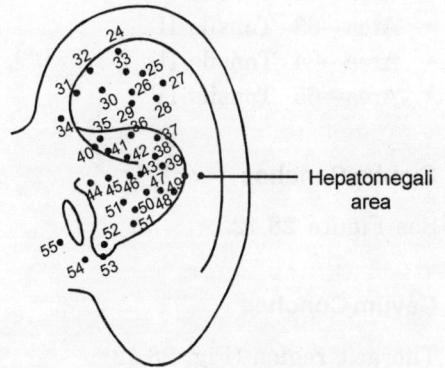

Figure 28.12: Points on triangular fossa, cavum conchae and cymba conchae

Helix

Genitals and Urethra are located.

Scapha

This area represents upper limb (Fig. 28.13)

- Area—56 Finger
- Area—57 Hand
- Area—58 Wrist
- Area—59 Elbow
- Area—60 Shoulder
- Area—61 Clavicle
- Area—62 Tonsils I
- Area—63 Tonsils II
- Area—64 Tonsils III
- Area—65 Tonsils IV

Cymba Conchae

See Figure 28.12.

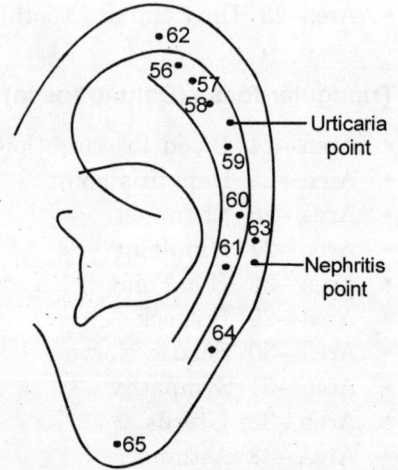

Figure 28.13: Points of scapha and helix

Cavum Conchae

Thoracic region (Fig. 28.12)

Cranial Surface of the Auricle

On the cranial surface of the auricle there is a groove, which corresponds to the antihelix. This is the lowering blood pressure groove. The remaining back of the auricle is divided to 3 areas upper, middle and lower which correspond to the area of the back and trunk. Back is divided into upper, middle and lower of the spinal cord is located at the higest point of the root of the auricle (spinal cord I) in front of the mastoid process (spinal cord II) at the lower margin of the root of the auricle (Fig. 28.14)

- Area—66 Spinal Cord I
- Area—67 Depression groove
- Area—68 Lower back
- Area—69 Middle back
- Area—70 Upper back
- Area—71 Spinal Cord II

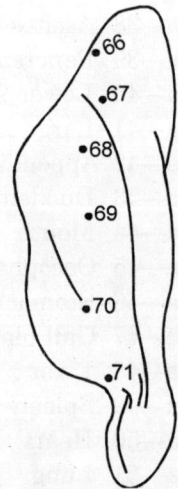

Figure 28.14: Points on the back of the auricle

Rules for the selection of the points

1. *Auricular points are of following categories*
   a. Those representing particular organs
   b. Those possessing special functions. AS
      i. Blood Pressure lowering point for hypertension
      ii. Shenmen for sedation
      iii. Endocrine point for hormonal regulation
      iv. Hot point for fever
   c. Specific point for disorders as
      i. Dingchan for asthma
      ii. Ascitis point for oedema
   d. In treating diseases, the points can be selected from above categories in various combination:
      i. Organ affected
      ii. Sedation point
      iii. Endocrine point
2. *Use of the meridian system*—Areas representing the pertaining organ can be used in the treatment of the diseases along the pathway of the meridian.
3. *Coupled organ*—For example small intestine for heart, spleen and gastric ulcer.
4. *Application* of the western knowledge of medicine, for example pancreas for diabetes mellitus.
5. *Use* of the point detector low electrical resistance point of the auricle.
6. *By examination* of the auricle through inspection and palpation.

Procedure

Fine filliform needles and press needles are inserted and stimulated by hand or with a high frequency electric current. Where prolonged stimulation of an acupuncture point is required, as in certain internal organ disorders, a small ear-press needle is left in situ (in its original place) for 7 to 10 days to obtain a better response. The ear press needles are circular in form, and about 3 mm in diameter with a tip which penetrate to a depth of 2-3 mm. These are left in place with an adhesive tape. In this period hand stimulation is not advisable.

SCALP ACUPUNCTURE (Head Needle Therapy)

Scalp Needling therapy was created by Chiao-Shun-Fa a Chinese physician. In his studies, he applied this therapy on the patient of cerebral stroke and paralysis he got positive results. This prompted him to discover other areas using the same technique.

It is a fact that the electrical field of the brain as projected on the scalp is acceptable to the western medical man since it forms the basis of EEG (Electro encephalo gram).

Thus, the relationship between brain areas and areas of scalp acupuncture is electro-physiological not topographical.

Indications for Scalp Acupuncture

1. Extrapyramidal disorders—Chorea, parkinsonism.
2. Post stroke hemiplegia
3. Intra cranial inflammation and their residual effects after the patient has recovered from coma
4. Spinal cord diseases as multiple sclerosis, urinary incontinence.
5. Intracranial parasites as cystitiserosis.
6. Peripheral nerve disorders as Trigeminal Neuralgia.
7. Psychological disorders—Nocturnal enuresis in children, impotency.
8. Myopathies as muscular atrophy.
9. Visceral diseases as gastric ulcer.
10. Cardiovascular disorders as, hypertension, bradycardia, tachycardia.
11. Speech disorders, as Asphasia, aphonia
12. Chest diseases as cough, asthma
13. Gynaecological disorders—as prolapse uterus.
14. Vestibulo—auditory disorders as vertigo, deafness, earache, tinnitus
15. Opthalmic disorders—as colour blindness
16. Acupuncture Anesthesia
17. Epilepsy

Division of the Areas

1. Main surface lines of the scalp
   Two imaginary lines are drawn
   i. Antero-posterior midline—It is the line connecting the mid point between the two eyebrows and the lower part of external occipital protuberance (Fig. 28.9)
   ii. Eyebrow—Occipit line—It is the line connecting the center of the eyebrow with the tip of the external occipital protuberance. It is drawn on the lateral aspect of the scalp (Fig. 28.15)
2. Localisation of the brain projection areas (Fig. 28.16)
   Area—1—Motor area
   i Lower 2/5 of the motor area represents for contralateral face.
   Indication—Motor aphasia, Aphasia, Aphonia, contra lateral central facial palsy
   ii Middle 2/5 of the motor area represent contralateral upper limb.
   Indication—Paralysis of contralateral arm
   iii Upper 1/5 of the motor area represent contralateral lower limb and trunk
   Indication—Paralysis of contralateral leg.
   Area 2—Sensory area
   i Upper 1/5 of the sensory area represents contralateral leg.
   Indication—parasthesia, sciatica, numbness.
   ii Middle 2/5 of the sensory area represents contralateral upper limb.
   Indication—Pain, numbness of contralateral arm.

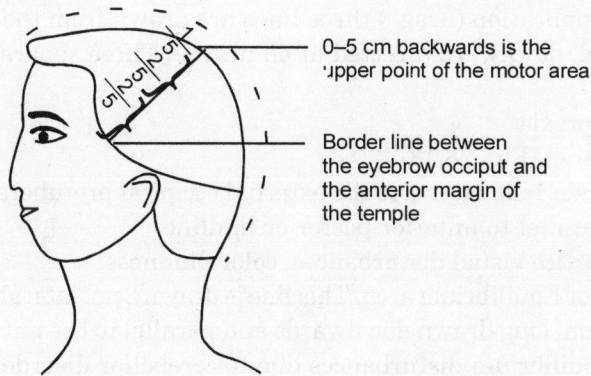

0–5 cm backwards is the upper point of the motor area

Border line between the eyebrow occiput and the anterior margin of the temple

Figure 28.15: Localisation of motor area

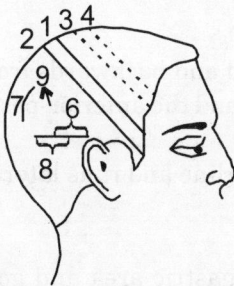

Figure 28.16: Scalp acupuncture area

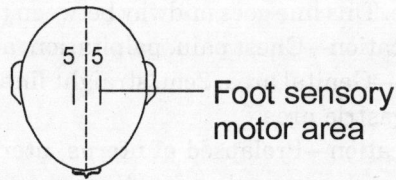

Foot sensory motor area

Figure 28.17: Surface of stimulation area

iii Lower 2/5 of the sensory area represent contralateral face.

Indication—Toothache, Trigeminal neuralgia, Contralateral facial numbness.

Area 3—Choreo—Tremor control area.

Indication—Senile tremors, parkinsonism, infantile chorea.

Area 4—Vasomotor area

Indication—Cerebral oedema, hypertension, hypotension.

Area 5—Foot sensory motor area (Fig. 28.17)

It runs 3 cm. Parallel to the anterior posterior midline.

Indication—Paralysis, numbness of the contralateral lower extremity, pain, acute pain or sprain of lumbar region.

Area 6—Vertigo auditory area

It is 4cm. Horizontal straight-line located 1.5cm. Vertically above auricle.

Indication—vertigo, deafness, tinnitus

Area 7—The second speech area it runs 3cm. straight-line situated 2cm. posterior—inferior to the parietal tubercle parallel to the anterior-posterior midline.

Area 8—The third speech area it runs backward from the midpoint of the area 6 (vertigo-auditory area) up to 4cm.

Indication—sensory aphasia

Area 9—Area of application (usage) three lines are drawn from the parietal tubercle, 3cm. forward, backward, downward directed at 40 degree. Three separate needles are used for treatment.

Indication—Appraxia

Area 10—Visual area (Fig. 28.18)`

This line is drawn 1cm. lateral to the external occipital protuberance of 4cm. long drawn upward and parallel to anterior-posterior midline.

Indication—Cortico visual disturbances, colorblindness.

Area 11-–Balance or Equilibrium area. This line is drawn 3cm. lateral to the external occipital protuberance of 4cm. long drawn downwards and parallel to the anterior-posterior midline.

Indication—Equilibrium disturbances due to cerebellar disorders.

Area 12 (Fig. 28.19)

Gastric area—It is a 2cm. lone line, starting directly above the pupil at hairline and runs backward and parallel to the anterior-posterior midline.

Indication—Gastric disorders.

Area 13—Thoracic cavity area. It runs 4cm. long forward and backwards from the natural hair line. This line goes midway between the gastric area and the anterior-posterior midline.

Indication—Chest pain, palpitation, asthma.

Area 14—Genital area. 2cm. straight line starts from hairline and runs lateral and parallel to the gastric area.

Indication—Prolapsed of uterus, uterine bleeding.

Area 15—Hepatocystic area. It runs straight from the gastric area and goes forward.

Indication—Gastric ulcer, chronic hepatitis

Technique of Manipulation

1. The treatment area should be sterilized with 75% alcohol and 2.5% iodine tincture.
2. Needles are 28-gange thick and 1 or 1 ½ inches long with a double spiral handle so that rotating movement can be done easily.
3. Needle is twisted in with frequency of more than 200 times per minute for 3 to 4 minutes. Leave the needle for 5 to 10 minutes repeat the procedure twice or thrice and withdraw the needle.

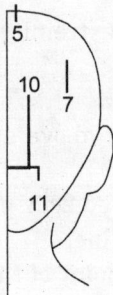

Figure 28.18: Posterior surface of the stimulation area

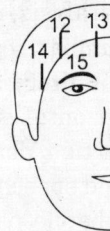

Figure 28.19: Anterior surface of the stimulation area

Hand and Foot Acupuncture

Hand

Hand acupuncture involves inserting needles at acupuncture points in the hand to cure various disease (Figs 28.20a and c).

- Area 1—Shoulder—It is located at lateral side of the metacarpophalangeal joint of the index finger.
  Indication—shoulder pain, frozen shoulder.
- Area 2—Forehead—It is located at first interphalangeal joint of the index finger.
  Indication—Frontal headache, sinusitis.
- Area 3—Vertex—It is located at lateral side of the first interphalangeal joint of the middle finger.
  Indication—Neurosis and headache.
- Area 4—Migraine—It is located at medical side of the first interphalangeal joint of the ring finger.
  Indication—Chest pain, migraine
- Area 5—Occipital—It is located at medical side of the first interphalangeal joint of the little finger.
  Indication—Occipital headache, pharyngitis, acute tonsillitis.
- Area 6—Sciatic nerve—It is located at medical side of the metacarpophalangeal joint of the ring finger.
  Indication—sciatica
- Area 7—Neck and Nape—It is located at medical side of the metacarpophalangeal joint of the index finger.
  Indication—Stiff neck, cervical spondylosis
- Area 8—Headache—It is located at medical side of the metacarpophalangeal joint of the thumb.
  Indication—Headache, dizziness
- Area 9—Nose—It is located at medical side of the metacarpal bone of the index finger.
  Indication—Nasal pain
- Area 10—Hysteria pain—It is located at center of the crease the metacarpophalangeal joint of the thumb
  Indication—Hysteria, psychosis, emotional disturbance.
- Area 11—Cough—It is located at medical side of the metacarpophalangeal joint of the index finger.
  Indication—Chronic bronchitis, asthma.
- Area 12—Oral ulcer—It is located at center of the crease of the metacarpophalangeal joint of the middle finger.
  Indication—Aphthous ulcers, Thrush.
- Area 13—Polyhidrosis—It is located at center of the palm
  Indication—Excessive sweating.
- Area 14—Liver—It is located at center of the first interphalangeal joint of the ring finger.
  Indication—Jaundice, Hepatitis

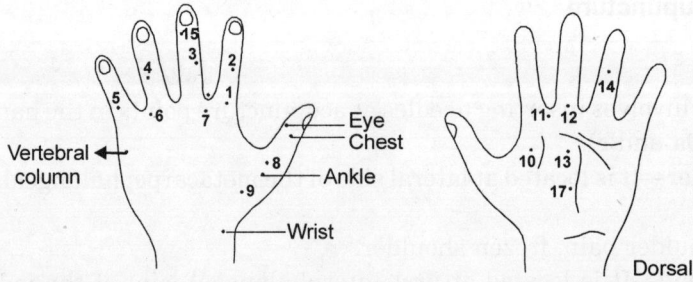

Figure 28.20 a and b: (a) Palmar surface and (b) dorsal surface

- Area 15—Hiccough—It is located at center of the second interphalangeal joint of the middle finger.
  Indication—hiccough
- Area 16—Antipyretic—It is located at lateral side of the web of the middle finger
  Indication—Pyrexia
- oArea 17—Anti-convulsion—It is located at junction of the thenar and hypothenar eminences in the palm.
  Indication—Febrile convulsions.

Foot (Figs 28.21a and b)

- Area 1—It is located between lateral and medical malleolus at sole
  Indication—Insomnia, hypertension, hysteria
- Area 2—It is located at 5-t-sun distal from posterior border of heal in the midline.
  Indication—Hepatitis
- Area 3—It is located at 1-t-sun proximal to the center of the 5th toe.
  Indication—Toothache
- Area 4—It is located at 2.5 t-sun below jiexi on dorsal aspect
  Indication—Angina pectoris
- Area 5—It is located at 1.5 t-sun proximal to the middle of the fourth and little toe.
  Indication—Sciatica
- Area 6—It is located at 2 t-sun proximal to the crease of the 3rd and 4th toe.
  Indication—Wry neck
- Area 7—It is located at medical side of the base of metatarsal bone of big toe.
  Indication—Loin pain
- Area 8—It is located at midway between xing jian and taichong.
  Indication—Tonsillitis

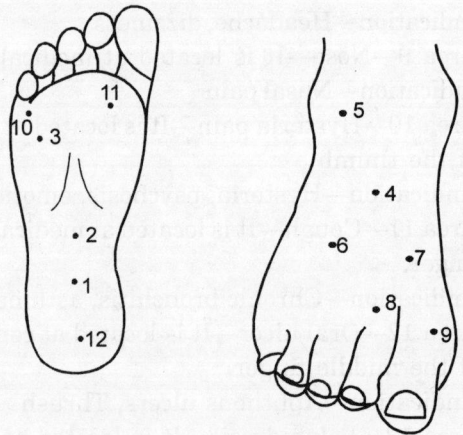

Figure 28.21 a and b

- Area 9—It is located at medical side of the tendon of the big toe.
  Indication—Eczema, Urticaria
- Area 10—It is located at middle of the metatarsophalangeal joint of little toe.
  Indication—Enuresis
- Area 11—It is located at 1 t-sun proximal to the middle of the web of big toe and the second toe at the planter aspect.
  Indication—Toothache
- Area 12—It is located at 1 t-sun distal to the posterior border of the heal at the midline
  Indication—Common cold.

NOSE AND FACE ACUPUNCTURE (Fig. 28.22)

This is very fine technique in which very fine cosmetic needles are inserted in the area of the nose and face.

There are three imaginary lines or the nose—one in the middle and two are located on the sides of the midline.

- First line—It is located in the middle it has acupuncture point for head and face, throat, lung, liver, heart, kidney and external genital organ. It is for solid or Yin organ
- Second Line—It is located at lateral to the midline, on both sides and has acupuncture point for gallbladder, small intestine, stomach, large intestine, bladder. It's for Hollow or YANG organs
- Third line—It is located at both lateral sides of the second line and has points for chest, breast, neck, ear, upper and lower extremities.

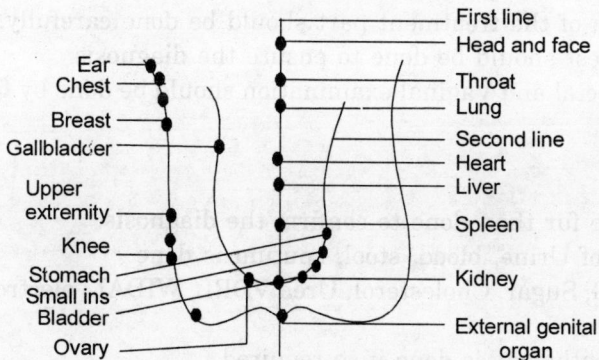

Figure 28.22: Nose acupuncture

chapter twenty-nine

Diagnosis

Diagnosis can be done either in (i) modern ways (ii) or traditional Chinese way.

MODERN DIAGNOSTIC METHOD

Like other general assessment first start with history of the patient. Except from name, age, sex ask for chief complaints, duration of illness occupation, living environment, social status, medical history.

Clinical Examination

We can examine in two ways
- General examination
- Systemic examination
  (i) General examination—Look for pulse, temperature, nails, glands, pupil, visible pulsations throat.
  (ii) Systemic examination—Look for digestive, Respiratory, Cardiovascular, genitourinary system. Musculoskeletal system.
  (iii) Local examination of the treatment part should be done carefully.
  (iv) Specific Clinical test should be done to ensure the diagnosis
  (v) Apart from this rectal and Vaginal examination should be done by finger and speculum.

Investigation

Investigation should be fur than done to confirm the diagnosis.
  (i) Laboratory tests of Urine, blood, stool, sputum is done
  (ii) X-rays, ECG, EEG, Sugar, Cholesterol, Urea VDRL, WIDAL, electromyogram is done in advanced stage.
  (iii) Biopsy and histopathology is done if so required.

TRADITIONAL CHINESE DIAGNOSTIC METHODS

  (i) Inspection—Inspect the patient in various ways as we do in modern times.
  (ii) Smell—Some disease can be diagnosed by smelling as coma and ketoacidisos
  (iii) Auscultation—Chinese were using their ear for Auscultation as stethoscope was not there.
  (iv) Percussion—Percussion were done as it is done in modern way.
  (v) Special test—These were done for eyes, tongue, lips, skin and nails.

(vi) Palpation—This is done in various ways
   - Pulse diagnosis
   - Palpation of whole body
   - Palpation of Ah-Shi points of particular area
(vii) History of dream—According to Chinese believe that dreams indicate present or future disease, but we require a specialist to analyse dreams.
(viii) This should be combined with patient's personal history, social history and past history.

PULSE DIAGNOSIS

According to the Chinese, for the successful diagnosis of a given disease, it is must to read the pulse.

Traditional Chinese medicine recognize 12 pulses. 6 pulses are on right wrist and 6 pulses are on left wrist.

Each has 3 superficial and 3 deep. The radial pulse is further divided in three section closer to wrist joint is called t-sun, cun, or inch (first position) middle is known as child or bar or guan (second position). Third is known as kuan or cubit or chih (third position). The superficial pulses are yang which can be felt by light touch and deep pulses are yin which can be felt by pressure.

Right wrist		Left wrist	
Deep	Superficial	Deep	Superficial
Pericardium	Triple warmer	Urinary bladder	Kidney
Spleen	Stomach	Gall bladder	Liver
Lung	Large intestine	Small intestine	Heart

Method of Pulse Diagnosis

- Physician should be Relaxed
- Silence should be maintained during diagnosis
- The best time is for pulse diagnosis is 5 am to 12 pm.
- Position of the patient
   a. Patient should be relaxed totally at least 5 to 10 minute before pulse diagnosis.
   b. Therapist should face the patient while taking pulse and a small cushion should be kept under wrist for slight dorsi flexion in order to relax, which makes the palpation much easier.
- In case of male, pulse is first taken in left wrist and in case of female pulse is first taken in right wrist.
- Therapist should place the tip of the index, middle and ring finger on the first, second and third position respectively of the Radial artery of one hand pulses are taken by therapist's right hand and the right wrist pulses from his left finger tips.

- After finishing the procedure make proper chart to have a proper record which further helps in proper diagnosis.

  The pulse of the left wrist is normally stronger than right wrist.

While pulse diagnosis look for

1. Pulse rate count the pulse beat, respiration per minute. Calculate pulse-respiration ratio.
2. Pulse rhythm—normal pulse is rhythmic in nature
3. Pulse volume—normal pulse is calm and free flowing in nature.
4. Pulse strength
5. Regularity of pulse
6. Pulse character—normal pulse is elastic with certain amount of tension
7. Effect of temperature, weather, time of the day, sex, age on pulse palpation.

Note: Rate and strength of the pulse play the most important role is diagnosis rest help in progress and prognosis.

chapter thirty

Complications and Contraindications

CONTRAINDICATIONS

1. It should not be used on certain area
    a. Umbilicus area
    b. Nipple and breast tissue
    c. External genitals
    d. Fontanelles in children
    e. Points overlying vulnerable structures.
2. It should not be used in following circumstances:
    a. Mechanical obstruction and frank surgical cases like strangulated hernia, intussueption, intestinal perforation, fracture, etc.
    b. Patient under the influence of alcohol, full stomach, empty stomach, coitus, heavy exertion, etc.
    c. Malignancy—Acupuncture can be used for relief from symptoms and complications of cancer but not as a cancer cure.
    d. Pregnancy—It may be lead to miscarriage or still birth, but it can be useful to treat vomiting and pain of childbirth.
    e. Patient with bleeding disorders.

COMPLICATIONS

Complications does not occur often but may arise due to improper techniques or carelessness.
1. Pain—In some patient it varies in different degrees. This can be due to swift insertion of needle, bad needle, nervous patient or bad posture adopted by patient or therapist.
2. Needle dystocia—After needle is inserted on the acupuncture point, sometimes muscle may become shift due to local spasm, in such case needle get fixed into the muscle. In this case, needle should be left in place for sometime massage or brisk stroking can be given around the needle in order to reduce the spasm, which makes removal of needle easier.
3. Bent Needle—In case needle get bent during insertion, don't rush to remove the needle without knowing the type of bending otherwise it may damage internal blood vessel.
4. Fainting—Nervousness, tiredness, hunger weakness, painful insertion of needles and excessive stimulation may lead to fainting.

In order to avoid these complications, patient should be relaxed and have proper posture. If patient faints, Needles should be removed immediately and first aid should be given.

5. Injury to Internal organs—Careless needling may lead to injury of Internal organs. Injury to external organs can be avoided by having proper knowledge of anatomical landmark, correct technique and controlling the depth and direction of needle insertion.

6. Infection—This can be avoided by paying attention to sterilization of needles and taking aseptic precautions while doing procedure.

7. Bleeding—While withdrawing needle sometimes bleeding may occur, which can be easily controlled by pressure on the point.

8. Forgotten needle—It is always advisable to count the needle before needling and recount them at the time of removal, otherwise left out needle can lead to infection and bleeding.

chapter thirty-one

Acupuncture Points

There are over 2,000 acupuncture points recognized by the Therapist and of these about 365 points, which are commonly used, are on the 14 main meridians

The acupuncture points can be classified in two ways.

i. Anatomically
ii. Functionally

Anatomical Classification

1. Meridian Points—The acupuncture point which goes the lines of the classical channels are known as meridian points. Their number is written with the short name of the channel. For example, SP-3 is the name given to third point on spleen, Liv-14 is fourteenth point on liver.
2. Extra meridian points—They are mainly on ear, nose, hand and head and they don't belong to old traditionally described points.
3. Floating points—They don't have any specific point. They exist on the diseased part and become tender or sensitive.

Functional Classification

Back-Shu Points **(Table 31.1)**

They are situated on the back of the urinary bladder channel.

Table 31.1: Back-Shu points

Sr.No.	Name	No.	Location	Related organ	Therapeutic use
1.	Jueyinshu	Ub-14	T-4	Pericardium	Pericarditis
2.	Ganshu	Ub-18	T-9	Liver	All liver disorder, backache
3.	Weishu	Ub-21	T-12	Stomach	All gstric disorder
4.	Feishu	Ub-13	T-3	Lung	Pneumonia, TB, bronchial asthma
5.	Xinshu	Ub-15	T-5	Heart	All cardiac problems
6.	Danshu	Ub-19	T-10	Gall bladder	Disorders of G.B.
7.	Pishu	Ub-20	T-11	Spleen	Allergy oedema
8.	Xiaochangshu	Ub-27	S-1	Small intestine	Disorders of S.I. sacro-iliac & lumbago
9.	Pangguangshu	Ub-28	S-2	Urinary bladder	Urine retention lumbosacral pain
10.	Shenshu	Ub-23	L-2	Kidney	Renal disorder genital disorder
11.	Sanjiaoshu	Ub-22	L-1	Triple warmer	Maintain homeostesis
12.	Dachangshu	Ub-25	L-4	Large intestine	Constipation, sciatica, low back pain

Yuan Points (Table 31.2)

They are used in the treatment of chronic disorders since these points possess maximum energy of the channel. These points are located around the ankle and wrist.

Table 31.2: Yuan points

Sr.No.	Name of the point	Name of the channel	Number
1.	Taixi	Kidney	K—3
2.	Hegu	Largeintestine	L1—4
3.	Taibai	Spleen	Sp—3
4.	Shenmen	Heart	H—7
5.	Taichong	Liver	Liv—3
6.	Chong Yang	Stomach	St—42
7.	Jinggu	Urinary Bladder	Ub—64
8.	Yangchi	Triple Warmer	Tw—4
9.	Handwangu	Small Intestine	S1—4
10.	Daling	Pericardium	P—7
11.	Taiyuan	Lung	L—9
12.	Qiuxu	Gall Bladder	Gb—40

Mu-front Points (Table 31.3)

They are situated on front of the chest and abdomen.

Distal Points

These points are situated on the specific distal part of the extremities and have therapeutic properties on the proximal part of the body

Extremity	Area of influence	Point
Upper Limb	Face, front of neck	Hegu (Li—4)
	Back of head	Lieque (L—7)
	Nape of neck	
	Back of chest	
	Front of chest and abdomen	Neiguan (P—6)
Lower Limb	Abdominal organ	Zusanli (St—36)
	Genital organ	Sanyinjao (Sp—6)
	Pelvic organ	Weizhong (Ub—40)
	Kidney	

Table 31.3: Mu-Front points

Sr. No.	Name	Number	Location	Related organ	Therapeutic uses
1.	Zhongfu	L-1	Inter space between the 1st & 2nd ribs.6t-Sun lateral to midline of chest	Lung	Bronchial asthma, Cough, Chest pain
2.	Tianshu	St-25	2t-Sun lateral to umbilicus	Large intestine	Paralytic Ileus, Costal pain, Abdominal distension
3.	Jujue	CV-14	6-T-Sun above the umbilicus in midline	Heart	Anxiety, Palpitation mental disorders
4.	Riyue	Gb-24	7th intercostal space	Gall bladder	Hepatitis
5.	Qimen	Liv-14	Below the nipple in 6th intercostal space	Liver	Chest pain, Pleuritis
6.	Jingmen	Gb-25	Free end of 12th rib	Kidney	Subcostal pain and Renal disorder
7.	Shimen	CV-5	2t-Sun below umbilicus in midline	Triple warmer	Irregular menstruation, Amenorrhoea, Oedema
8.	Zhangmen	Liv-13	Free end of 11th rib	Spleen	Pain in subcostal region, Diarrhoea
9.	Guanyuan	CV-4	3t-Sun below umbilicus in midline	Small intestine	Menorrhagia, Menstrual dysfunction impotence
10.	Shanzhong	CV-17	Midway between the two nipples	Pericardium	Bronchial asthma Chest pain, Bronchitis
11.	Zhongji	CV-3	4t-Sun below umbilicus in midline	Urinary bladder	Pelvic Inflammation, Urine retention, Incontinence of urine
12.	Zhongwan	CV-12	Midway between umblicus and xiphoid process	Stomach	Dyspepsia, Gastritis, Vomiting

Confluent Points

There are eight points on the twelve meridians in the extremities. They are as follow—

Houxi	-	SI—3	
Waiguan	-	TW—5	
Gongsun	-	SP—4	
Zhaohai	-	K—6	
Foot Linqi	-	GB—41	
Lieque	-	L—7	
Neiguan	-	P—6	
Shenmai	-	UB—62	

Tonification Points

All the twelve meridians have a point when these points are stimulated bring the tonification of the meridian. For example, Fuliu (K—7) is stimulated tonification of the kidney occurs.

They are as follow

Quchi	- (LI—11)	Zhongchong	(P—9)
Jiexi	- (St—41)	Zhiyin	(UB—67)
Fuliu	- (K—7)	Zhongzhu	(TW—3)
Xiaxi	- (GB—43)	Shao-Chong	(H—9)
Ququan	- (Liv—8)	Dadu	(SP—2)
Taiyuan	- (L—9)	Quyuan	(SI—13)

Sedation Points

These points when stimulated gives sedative effect to meridians.

Example—Shugu (UB—65) being the point of sedation for the urinary bladder when it is stimulated brings sedation to urinary bladder meridian.

Lidui	- (St—45)
Xiaohai	- (SI—8)
Shugu	- (UB—65)
Rangu	- (K—2)
Tianjing	- (TW—10)
Daling	- (P—7)
Erjian	- (LI—2)
Sanjian	- (LI—3)
Chize	- (l—5)
Shangqiu	- (SP—5)
Yangungquam	- (GB—34)
Xingjian	- (Liv—2)
Yongquan	- (K—1)

Jing-Well Point

These points can be stimulated in acute emergencies like cardiac failure, shock. Almost all the points are located on toes and fingers near nail bed.

Alarm Point

These point's works as alarm signals as they become painful or tender in the disorder of respective organ. These points can be used for diagnosis, treatment, and prognosis.

Luo-Connecting Points

These points are the connecting links between YIN and YANG channels. The advantages of Luo-connecting points are when given treatment.

a. Only one connecting point controls the energy between the left and right halves of a meridian.

b. Only one point can bring equilibrium in two luo-connected meridians.

Dangerous Points

These points are in the close vicinity of vital organ, they are known as dangerous points. Example—Chengqui (St—1) is located near eye; it is likely to damage during needling.

Influential Points

Eight important tissues of the body are influenced by eight different points. Diseases of these tissues can be treated by combining them with other point.

Blood	- Geshu	(UB—17)
Bone	- Dashu	(UB—11)
Bone marrow	- Xuanzhong	(GB—39)
Blood Vessels	- Taiyuan	(L—9)
Muscle & Tendon	- Yanglingquan	(GB—34)
Respiratory tissue	- Shanzhong	(CV—17)
Solid Organs	- Zhangmen	(Liv—13)
Hallow organs	- Zhongwan	(CV—12)

chapter thirty-two

Meridian System

According to traditional Chinese theory, 12 paired meridians, Meridians running vertically from below upward or above downwards are main meridians. The 12 paired meridians originated from the internal viscera of the body and are named according to the viscera of origin.

The twelve main meridians are-
1. The heart meridian(H)
2. The small intestine meridian(SI)
3. The bladder meridian(U-BL)
4. The kidney meridian(K)
5. The pericardium meridian(P)
6. The Triple warmer meridian(TW)
7. The gall bladder meridian(GB)
8. The Liver meridian(LI)
9. The Lung meridian(L)
10. The spleen meridian(SP)
11. The stomach meridian(SI)
12. The large intestine meridian(LI)

THE HEART MERIDIAN (Fig. 32.1)

The heart meridian is a Yin meridian. It receives energy from spleen meridian. *Location* -starting point is located under the pectoralis muscle at the level of 3rd rib. It runs alongside and inside of the upper and lower arm and ends on inside of the distal section of the little finger. It connects with the small intestine channel. The heart meridian runs in a centrifugal direction.

The heart meridian has 9 points.

H-1

Location—Centre of axilla, medial to axillary artery
Indication—Shoulder pain, Brachial neuralgia, upper limb paralysis, pain in arm.

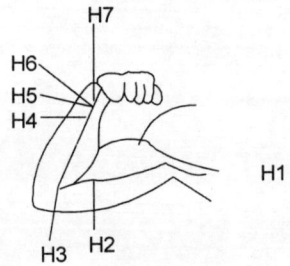

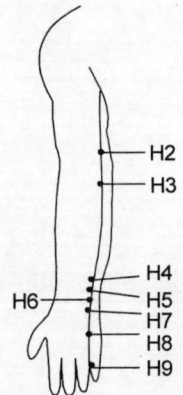

Figure 32.1: The heart meridian

H-2

Location—Antero-medial aspect of arm in a groove medial to the biceps brachii, 3 t-sum above elbow.
Indication—Shoulder and Arm pain, Costal and subcostal pain

H-3

Location—Midpoint of the line joining medial end of the transverse cubital crease and medial epicondyle of the humerus, when elbow is flexed.
Indication—Arthritis of elbow, tennis elbow, tremor and numbness of the arm.

H-4

Location—Medial aspect to forearm, 1.5 t-sun above the posterior border of pisiform bone, lateral to tendon of flexor carpi ulnaris
Indication—Ulna neuralgia, Arthritis of wrist joint

H-5

Location—1-t-sun above the posterior border of the pisiform bone, lateral to flexor carpi Ulnaris tendon.
Indication—Insomnia, painful arm and wrist, aphasia

H-6

Location—On front of wrist, 0.5 t-sun proximal to the posterior border of the pisiform bone lateral to the flexor carpi ulnaris tendon.
Indication—Angina pectoris, MI, Neurasthenia.

H-7

Location—Proximal to pisiform bone in a groove lateral to the flexor carpi ulnaris tendon.
Indication—Epilepsy, Palpitation, Hysteria

H-8

Location—On the palm between the 4th and 5th metacarpal bones.
Indication—Carpal tunnel syndrome, Arthritis of carpal joint. Chest pain, Palpitation, costalgia.

H-9

Location—On the lateral side of the little finger about 0.1 t-sun proximal to the lateral corner of the nail.
Indication—Chest pain, coronary thrombosis, coma.

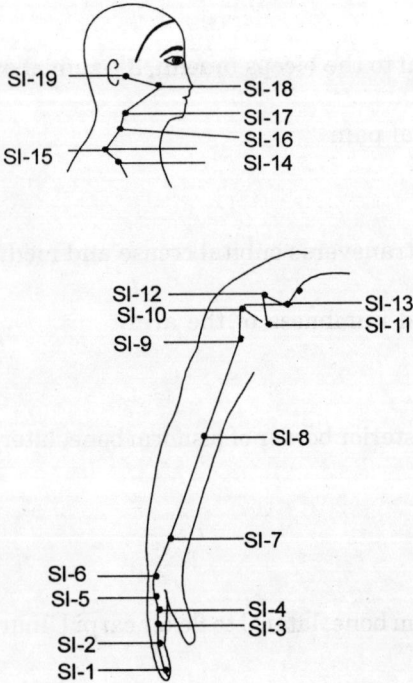

Figure 32.2a: Small intestinal meridian

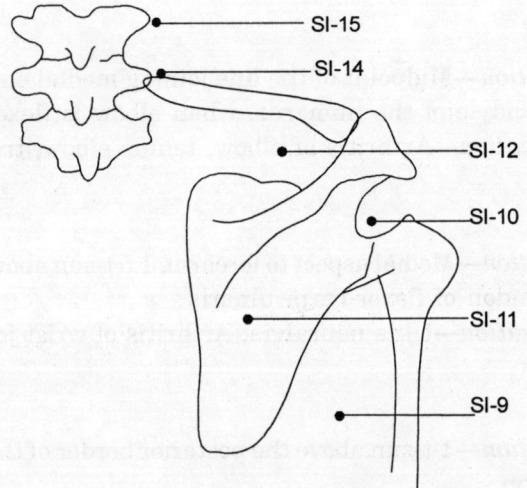

Figure 32.2b: Small intestine meridian

THE SMALL INTESTINE MERIDIAN (Figs 32.2a and b)

The small intestinal meridian is a yang meridian, which receives its energy from heart meridian. It's maximum time lies between 13 to 15 hrs. This is the best time for sedating treatment. It is better to tonify after this time. This meridian has starting point at the ulna angle at the nail on the little finger, going up along the ulna border of the hand to the elbow. It then goes via the dorsal side of the upper arm and shoulder blade to the neck and then it runs to the cheekbone to the hollow of the tragus in front of the ear.

SI-1

Location—0.1 t-sun proximal to the corner of the nail of the little finger on its medial side.
Indication—Shock, Convulsion, All acute emergencies like respiratory and cardiac arrest.

SI-2

Location—On the ulnar side of the metacarpophalangeal joint of the little finger
Indication—Tingling and numbness of the fingers, painful arm, diminished vision.

SI-3

Location—At the medial end of the main transverse palmar crease, on the ulnar border of the hand, Proximal to the 5th metacarpophalangeal joint.
Indication—Stiffness of the neck, cervical spondylosis, paralysis of upper limb, epilepsy.

SI-4

Location—On the ulna border of the hand between the 5th metacarpal bone and the hamate bone.
Indication—Wrist arthritis, Stiffness of fingers, wrist drop. Headache.

SI-5

Location—On the medial aspect of the wrist in a groove between the posiform bone and the ulnar styloid process
Indication—Pain in wrist, cervical pain, cervical spondylosis, deafness.

SI-6

Location—On the posterior aspect of the wrist in a groove lateral to the ulnar styloid process, proximal to the inferior radio-ulnar joint.
Indication—upper limb paralysis, wrist arthritis, wrist-drop, stiff neck, cervical spondylosis.

SI-7

Location—On the ulnar side of the forearm 5t-sun proximal to SI-5
Indication—Stiff neck, cervical spondylosis

SI-8

Location—In a depression on the back of the elbow between olecranon and medial epicondyle.
Indication—Stiff neck, elbow and shoulder pain, ulnar neuritis

SI-9

Location—1 t-sun above the lower margin of the posterior axillary fold
Indication—Shoulder joint periarthritis, paralysis and polyneuropathy of the upper limb.

SI-10

Location—Vertically above SI-9 just below the spine of scapula
Indication—Periarthritis of shoulder, paralysis of upper limb.

SI-11

Location—At the level with the Spinous process of the 4th thoracic vertebra, in the center of infra-scapular fossa.
Indication—Painful conditions of upper limb.

SI-12

Location—At the center of infrascapular fossa
Indications—Shoulder pain, Numbness of upper limb.

SI-13

Location—In the suprascapular fossa, near the medical border of the scapula midway between the spinous process of second thoracic vertebra and SI-10.
Indication—Pain and Contracture of shoulder joint, Restricted movement.

SI-14

Location—3-t sun lateral to the inferior border of the spinous process of the 1st thoracic vertebra.
Indication—Cervical spondylosis, pain in the back of the shoulder and scapula, stiff neck.

SI-15

Location—2 t-sun lateral to the inferior border of the spinous process of the 7th cervical vertebra.
Indication—Frozen shoulder, Myositis and muscle cramps.

SI-16

Location—On the posterior border of the sterno-cleido-mastoid muscle at the level with the laryngeal prominence.
Indication—Cervical spondylosis, Neck stiffness, Sore throat, Painful tonsil.

SI-17

Location—Behind the angle of the jaw on the anterior border of the sterno-cleido-mastoid muscle.
Indication—Tonsillitis, Sore throat.

SI-18

Location—Below the inferior border of the Zygomatic bone at a level vertically below the outer canthus of the eye.
Indication—Bells' Palsy, Facial muscle, Spasm, Trigeminal neuralgia.

SI-19

Location—In the depression between the tragus of the ear and temporomandibul joint when the mouth is slightly open.
Indication—Arthritis of temporomandibular joint, deafness, otitis media.

THE KIDNEY MERIDIAN (Figs 32.3a to d)

The kidney meridian is a yin meridian which receives its energy from the bladder meridian. It's maximum time lies between 17 to 19 hours which is the best time for a sedating treatment. The meridian starts at the sole of the foot, goes inside the foot, travels a circle behind and in front of the malleous internus lower leg and the thigh upto bladder passes naval and breast bone ending on the sternal side of clavicle. It has 27 points.

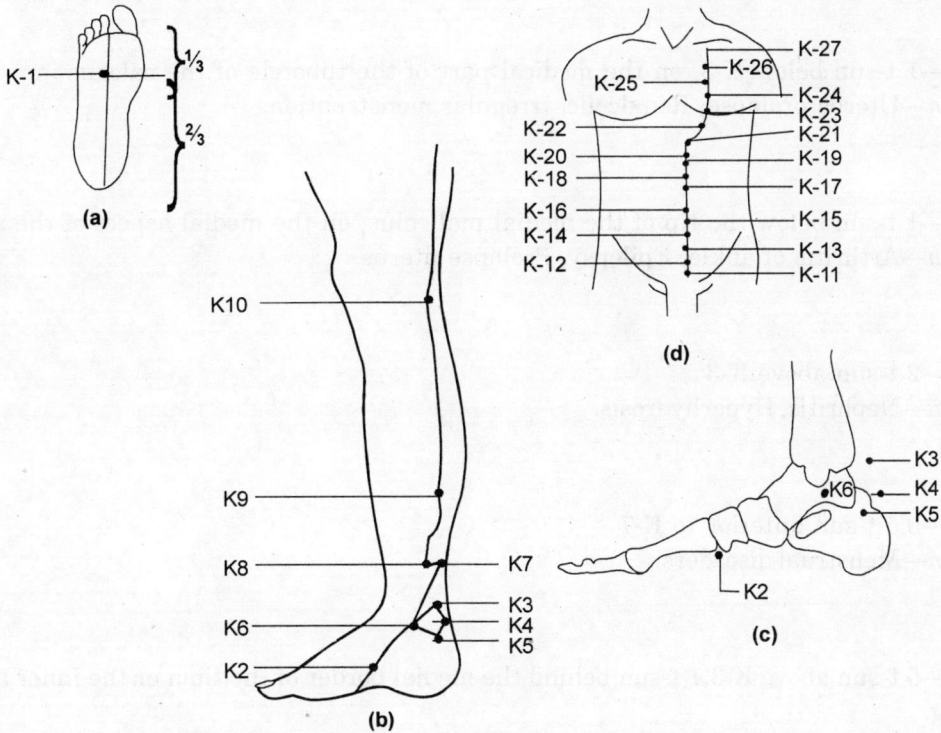

Figures 32.3a to d: The kidney meridian

K-1

Location—In the hollow of the sole at the junction of it's anterior 1/3 and posterior 2/3 in the depression between the 2nd and 3rd metatarsophalangeal joints.
Indication—Unconsciousness, Epilepsy, Foot drop, Foot arthritis, Planter fascitis.

K-2

Location—On the medial border of the foot in the depression. Postero-inferior to the tuberosity of the navicular bone.
Indication—Menorrhagia, Planterfascitis, Diabetes, Cystitis.

K-3

Location—Midway between the tip of medial malleous and tendo-achilles.
Indication—Foot drop, Planterfascitis, Calcanear spur, Paralysis of lowerlimb, Urinary incontinence, Nephritis.

K-4

Location—Posterior-inferior to K-3 in front of the tendo-achilles and above the calcaneus.
Indication—Asthma, Constipation, Calcaneal spur, Planter fascitis.

K-5

Location—1 t-sun below K-3, on the medical part of the tubercle of the calcaneum.
Indication—Uterus prolapse, Renalcolic, Irregular menstruation.

K-6

Location—1 t-sun below the tip of the medial malleolus, on the medial aspect of the ankle.
Indication—Arthritis of ankle, Epilepsy, Prolapse uterus.

K-7

Location—2 t-sun above K-3
Indication—Nephritis, Hyperhydrosis.

K-8

Location—0.5 t-sun anterior to K-7
Indication—Menstrual disorders.

K-9

Location—5 t-sun above K-3.1 t-sun behind the medial border of the tibia or the inner aspect of the leg.
Indication—Calf muscle cramp, Epilepsy.

K-10

Location—At the medial side of Popliteal fossa, between tendon of semitendinosus and semi-membranous.
Indication—Painful knee conditions, Genital problems.

K-11

Location—In the lower abdomen 0.5 t-sun lateral to CV-2
Indication—Urine incontinence, Impotence, Dysuria, Vaginal prolaps, Painful red eye.

K-12

Location—1 t-sun directly above K-11 and 0.5 t-sun lateral to CV-3.
Indication—Vulvitis, Leucorrhoea, Spermatorrhoea flour albus.

K-13

Location—2 t-sun directly above K-11 and 0.5 t-sun lateral to CV-4.
Indication—Menstrual disorders, Diarrhoea, Pain at postpartum, eyes infection.

K-14

Location—3 t-sun directly above K-11.
Indication—Same as K-13.

K-15

Location—0.5 t-sun lateral to CV-7.
Indication—Menstrual disorders, lower abdomen pain.

K-16

Location—0.5 t-sun lateral to umbilicus.
Indication—Menstrual disorders, Hernia, Jaundice, Constipation.

K-17

Location—2-t sun directly above K-16, and 0.5 t-sun lateral to midline.
Indication—Anorexia, Hiatus hernia.

K-18

Location—3 t-sun directly above K-16 and 0.5 t-sun lateral to the midline.
Indication—Constipation, Epigastric Pain, Hiccup.

K-19

Location—4 t-sun above K-16 and 0.5 t-sun lateral to the midline.
Indication—Epigastric Pain.

K-20

Location—5 t-sun above K-16 and 0.5 t-sun lateral to midline.
Indication—Epigastric Pain, Gastralgia, Abdominal distension.

K-21

Location—6 t-sun above K-16 and 0.5 t-sun lateral to midline.
Indication—Constriction of chest, Belching or Diarrhoea, Nausea, Upper abdomen pain.

K-22

Location—On the front of the chest in the 5th intercostal space, 2 t-sun lateral to the midline.
Indication—Pleuritis, Pleurisy, Intercostal neuralgia, Bronchitis.

K-23

Location—On the front of the chest in the 4th intercostal space, 2 t-sun lateral to CV-17.
Indication—Same as K-22.

K-24

Location—3rd intercostal space, 2 t-sun lateral to midline.
Indication—Vomiting, Bronchitis, Thoracalgia.

K-25

Location—2nd intercostal space, 2 t-sun lateral to midline.
Indication—Bronchitis, Intercostal neuralgia, Cough.

K-26

Location—1st intercostal space 2 t-sun lateral to the midline, midway between the sternal and mammilary lines.
Indication—Bronchitis, Thoracalgia, Cough.

K-27

Location—In the hollow between the lower border of the clavicle and the 1st rib, 2 t-sun lateral to the midline.
Indication—Thoracalgia, Bronchitis, Cough, Asthma, Painful chest.

THE BLADDER MERIDIAN

The bladder meridian as a Yang meridian which obtains it's energy from the small intestine meridian. It's maximum time lies between 15 hrs to 17 hrs. which is the best time for a sedating treatment. Tonification is better after this time.

This is the longest channel. It begins at the medial canthus of the eye, runs over the forehead and head close to the midline, where it divides into two branches at the 2nd cervical vertebra. The medial branch runs at a distance of 1 1\2 CUN along side the meridian line. The 2nd branch runs at 1 1\2 CUN more lateral than the 1st branch. And they cross each other descend down up to the back of the popliteal fossa, where they unite in the middle to form a single branch. This single main branch runs down on the back of the leg and lateral border of the foot and ends at the lateral aspect of the tip of the little toe.

It has 67 points.

U-BL-1 (Fig. 32.4a)

Location—On the margin of the orbit 0.1 t-sun above the medial canthus.
Indication—Myopia, atrophy, facial paralysis, conjunctivitis, opticneuralgia.

NOTE: It a dangerous point, extra care should be taken while needling.

U-BL-2

Location—At the inner end of the eyebrow directly above the inner canthus of the eye.
Indication—Frontal sinusitis, trigeminal neuralgia, eye and nose disease.

U-BL-3 (Figs 32.4b and c)

Location—Above U-BL –2, 0.5 t-sun inside the natural hair line
Indication—Headache, blurring of vision.

U-BL-4 (Fig. 32.4c)

Location—1.5 t-sun lateral and 0.5 t –sun inside the midpoint of the anterior natural hair line.
Indication—Frontal sinusitis, headache, nasal congestion.

U-BL-5

Location— 1 t-sun above anterior natural hairline. Above BL-4.
Indication—Epilepsy, frontal headache, and sinusitis.

U-BL-6

Location—1.5 t-sun behind BL-5.
Indication—Headache, dizziness.

U-BL-7

Location—3 t-sun behind BL-5
Indication—Same as BL-6

U-BL-8

Location—4.5 behind BL-5.
Indication—Nasal congestion, nose bleeding, vertical headache.

U-BL-9 (Fig. 32.4d)

Location—1.3 t-sun lateral to the midpoint of the superior border of the external occipital protuberance.
Indication—Occipital headache, myopia, giddiness

U-BL-10

Location—On the lateral side of the trapezius 0.5 t –above the natural hair line 0.3 t-sun lateral to midline between the 1st and 2nd cervical vertebrae.
Indication—Epilepsy, occipital headache, insomnia, neck stiffness.

U-BL-11

Location—On the back 1.5 t—sun lateral to the tip of the spinous process of the 1st thoracic vertebra.
Indication—Asthma, arthritis and numbness of limb, backache, neckpain, bronchitis, pneumonia, pleurisy.

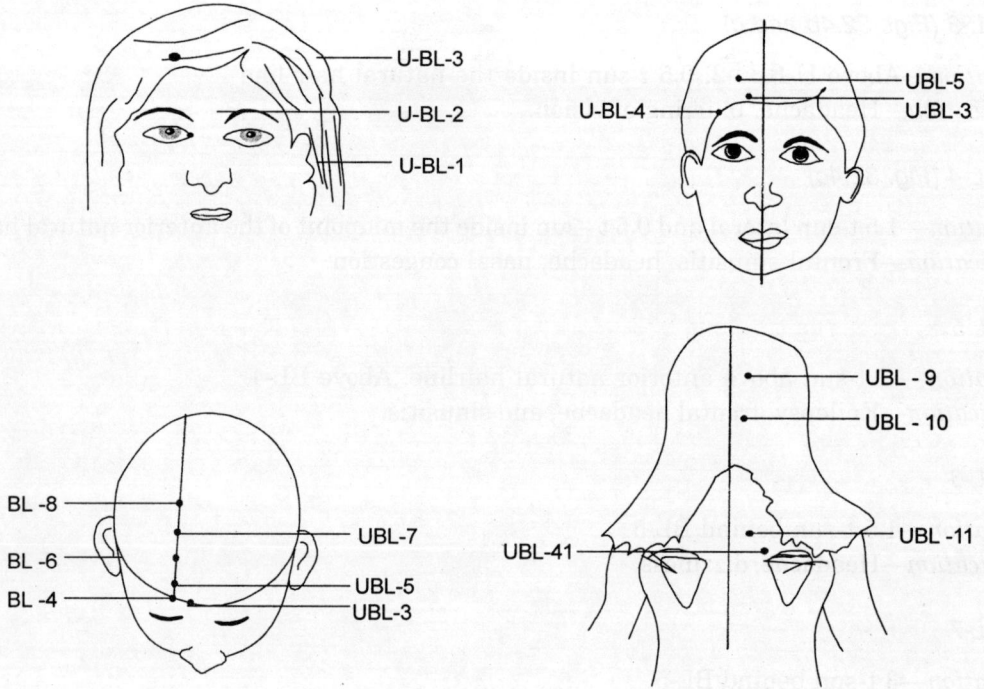

Figure 32.4a to d: Bladder meridian

U-BL-12 (Fig. 34.4e)

Location—On the back 1.5 t –sun lateral to the tip of the spinous process of the 2nd thoracic vertebrae.
Indication—Allergy, bronchitis.

U-BL-13

Location—On the back 1.5 t-sun lateral to the tip of the spinous process of the 3rd thoracic vertebra and with the level of spine of scapula.
Indication—Asthma, cough, cold, low back pain, tuberculosis, bronchitis.

Note: It is an alarm point for lung.

U-BL-14

Location—On the back, 1.5 t-sun lateral to the tip of spinous process of the 4th thoracic vertebra.
Indication—Chest pain, palpitation, mental disorders.

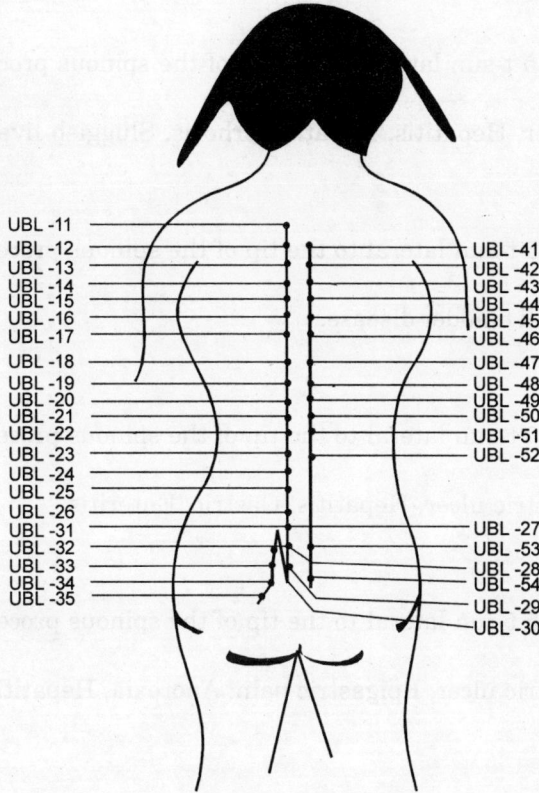

Figure 32.4e

U-BL-15

Location—On the back, 1.5 t-sun lateral to the tip of the spinous process of the 5th thoracic vertebra.
Indication—Palpitation, epilepsy, memory loss.

U-BL-16

Location—On the back 1.5 t-sun lateral to the tip of the spinous process of the 6th thoracic vertebra
Indication—Abdominal pain, alopecia, endocarditis.

U-BL-17

Location—On the back, 1.5 t-sun lateral to the tip of the spinous process of the 7th thoracic vertebra at the level with the inferior angle of Scapula.
Indication—Diaphragm paralysis, Anorexia nerveosa, Anemia, Haemorrahagic disorders, Hiccup.

U-BL-18

Location—On the back 1.5 t-sun lateral to the tip of the spinous process of the 9th thoracic vertebra.
Indication—Alcoholic liver, Hepatitis, Hepatic cirrhosis, Sluggish liver.

U-BL-19

Location—On the back 1.5 t-sun lateral to the tip of the spinous process of the 10th thoracic vertebra.
Indication—Hepatitis, Gall bladder disease.

U-BL-20

Location—On the back 1.5 t-sun lateral to the tip of the spinous process of the 11th thoracic vertebra.
Indication—Oedema, Gastric ulcer, Hepatitis, Gastric, Enteritis.

U-BL-21

Location—On the back 1.5 t-sun lateral to the tip of the spinous process of the 12th thoracic vertebra.
Indication—Gastric, Gastric ulcer, Epigastric pain, Anorexia, Hepatitis.

U-BL-22

Location—On the back of abdomen 1.5 t-sun lateral to the tip of the spinous process of the 1st lumbar vertebra.
Indication—Same as BL-21, Lambago, Urine incontinence.

U-BL-23

Location—On the back of abdomen 1.5 t-sun lateral to the tip of the spinous process of the 2nd lumbar vertebra.
Indication—Lumbago, Impotence, Irregular menstruation, Nephritis, Genital disorders.

U-BL-24

Location—On the back of abdomen 1.5 t-sun lateral to the tip of the spinous process of the 3rd lumbar vertebra.
Indication—Prolapsed rectum, Lumbago.

U-BL-25

Location—On the back of abdomen 1.5 t-sun lateral to the tip of the spinous process of the 4th lumbar vertebra.
Indication—Constipation, Lumbago, Sciatica, Paralysis of lower limb.

U-BL-26

Location—On the back of abdomen 1.5 t-sun lateral to the tip of the spinous process of the 5th lumbar vertebra.
Indication—Lumbago, Urinary incontinence, Cystitis.

U-BL-27

Location—On the back of abdomen 1.5 t-sun lateral to the midline at the level of sacroiliac joint.
Indication—Sciatica, Lumbago, Urinary incontinence, Pelvic peritonitis.

U-BL-28

Location—1.5 t-sun lateral to the posterior midline over the sacroiliac at the level with the 2nd sacral vertebra.
Indication—Lumbo-sacral pain, sciatica, constipation, cystitis, ischia, urine incontence.

U-BL-29

Location—At the level of 3rd sacral vertebra, 1.5 t-sun lateral to the posterior midline.
Indication—Sciatica, sacroiliac pain, lumbosacral pain.

U-BL-30

Location—1.5 t-sun lateral to the posterior midline at the level with the hiatus sacralis
Indication—Sacral neuralgia, sciatica.

U-BL-31 (Fig. 32.4f)

Location—On the 1st posterior sacral foramen midway between the posterior midline and the posterior superior iliac spine.
Indication—Prolapsed rectum, menstrual disturbance, lumbago, hot flushes, headache, haemorrhoids, dysurea.

U-BL-32

Location—On the 2nd posterior sacral foramen midway between the lower part of the posterior superior iliac spine and the posterior midline
Indication—Urogenital disorders, lumbago, sciatica, menstrual disorder

U-BL-33

Location—On the third posterior foramen
Indication—Same as BL-32.

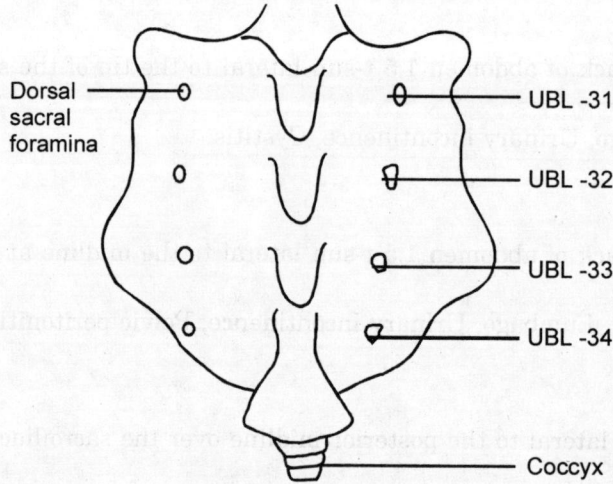

Figure 32.4f

U-BL-34

Location—On the forth posterior sacral foramen.
Indication—Same as BL-32

U-BL-35

Location—0.5 t-sun lateral to the posterior midline at
the level of tip of the coccyx.
Indication—Backache during menstrual period, lumbar
pain, impotence, leucorrhoea, diarrhoea.

U-BL-36 (Fig. 32.4g)

Location—Midpoint of the gluteal sulcus.
Indication—Sciatica, low back pain, paralysis of upper
limb, arthritis of hip joint.

U-BL-37

Location—6 t-sun below BL-36 in the center of the posterior aspect of thigh.
Indication—Low back ache, sciatica, lower limb paralysis.

U-BL-38

Location—On the lateral side of the popliteal fossa 1 t-sun above BL-39.
Indication—Constipation, poliomyelitis.

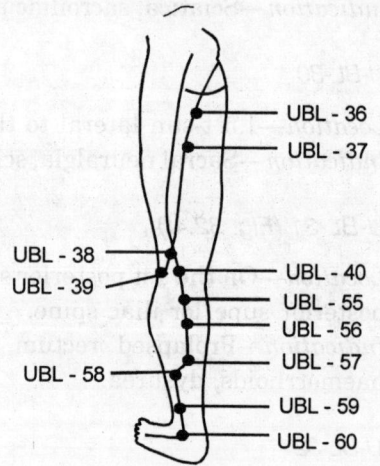

Figure 32.4g

U-BL-39

Location—On the lateral end of the popliteal crease, medial to biceps femoris tendon
Indication—Calf muscle cramp, low backache, paralysis of lower limb.

U-BL-40

Location—Midpoint of the popliteal fossa.
Indication—Lumabo, low back pain, sciatica, exzema, acne, knee arthritis, sunburn, genito-urinary disorders.

U-BL-41

Location—On the back 3 t-sun lateral to the tip of the spinous process of the 2nd thoracic vertebra.
Indication—Shoulder pain, frozen shoulder, inter costal neuralgia, numbness of elbow and arm.

U-BL-42

Location—On the back 3 t-sun lateral to the tip of the spinous process of the 3rd thoracic vertebra.
Indication—Bronchitis, asthma, pulmonary tuberculosis.

U-BL-43

Location—On the back 3- t sun lateral to the tip of the spinous process of the 4th thoracic vertebra.
Indication—Pulmonary tuberculosis, bronchitis.

U-BL-44

Location—On the back 3t-sun lateral to the tip of the spinous process of the 5th thoracic vertebra.
Indication—Heart disorders, frozen shoulder, backache.

U-BL-45

Location—On the back 3t-sun lateral to the tip of the spinous process of the 6th thoracic vertebra.
Indication—Inter costal neuralgia, asthma, bronchitis, vertigo.

U-BL-46

Location—On 3t-sun lateral to the tip of the spinous process of the 7th thoracic vertebra
Indication—Intercostal neuralgia, backache, belching.

U-BL-47

Location—On the back 3t-sun lateral to the tip of the spinous process of the 9th thoracic vertebra.
Indication—Hepatic disorder, epigastric pain.

U-BL-48

Location—On the back 3t-sun lateral to the tip of the spinous process of the 10th thoracic vertebra.
Indication—Jaundice, abdominal pain, hepatic disorders.

U-BL-49

Location—On the back 3t-sun lateral to the tip of the spinous process of the 11th thoracic vertebra.
Indication—Backache, flatulence, vomiting.

U-BL-50

Location—On the back 3t-sun lateral to the tip of the spinous process of the 12th thoracic vertebra.
Indication—Spinal pain, constipation, flatulence.

U-BL-51

Location—On the back of abdomen 3 t-sun lateral to the spinous process of the 1st lumbar vertebra.
Indication—Constipation, epigastric pain.

U-BL-52

Location—On the back of abdomen 3t-sun lateral to the spinous process of the 2nd lumbar vertebra.
Indication—Impotence, oedema, backache, phosphaturia.

U-BL-53

Location—On the dorsal surface of sacram 3t-sun lateral to the midpoint of the 2nd sacral vertebra.
Indication—Urine retention, backache, abdominal distension.

U-BL-54

Location—3t-sun lateral to the posterior midline at the level of the 4th sarcal foramen on the dorsal aspect of the sacrum.
Indication—Sciatica, sacroiliac pain, lower limb paralysis, low back pain, arthritis of hip joint, numbness and pain of lower limb.

U-BL-55

Location—2t-sun below BL-40
Indication—Lumbago, lower limb paralysis, leg cramp, polio.

U-BL-56

Location—Midway between BL-55 and BL-57
Indication—Same as BL-55.

U-BL-57.

Location—On the calf, where the tendon of gastronemius unite, midway between BL-40 and the heel
Indication—Sciatica, lower limb paralysis, planter fascitis, haemorrhoids, anus prolapse.

U-BL-58

Location—7t-sun above BL-60.
Indication—Sciatica, nephritis.

U-BL-59

Location—3t-sun above BL-60
Indication—Lumbosacral pain, headache, strain and arthritis of ankle joint.

U-BL-60 (Fig. 32.4h)

Location—Central part of the groove between the tendo achillis and posterior border of the lateral malleolus of the fibula at tip.
Indication—Foot drop, sciatica, low back ache, calcaneal spur, painful disorder of ankle, lower limb paralysis. Polio.

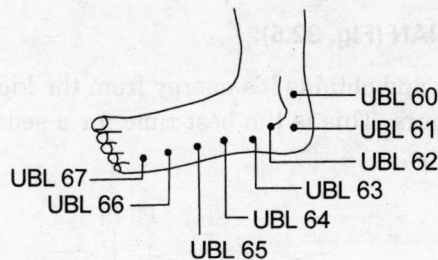

Figure 32.4h

U-BL-61

Location—1.5 t-sun below B-L-60
Indication—Calcaneal spur, painful heel, lowerlimb paralysis, ankle pain, planter fascitis.

U-BL-62

Location—On the outer aspect of ankle, 0.5 t-sun below the tip of the lateral malleolus.
Indication—Ankle pain, low backache, lowerlimb paralysis, foot drop, headache, insomnia.

U-BL-63

Location—Anterio–inferior to BL-62, proximal to the tuberosity of the 5th metatarsal bone
Indication—Infantile convulsion, ankle pain, epilepsy.

U-BL-64

Location—On the outer aspect of the foot, inferior to the tuberosity of the 5th metatarsal, at the junction of the two colors of skin.
Indication—Legpain, headache, epilepsy

U-BL-65

Location—On the lateral border of the foot, behind and below the 5th metatarsophalangeal joint.
Indication—Headache, vertigo, leg cramp, lumbago, pain along the lateral border of foot.

U-BL-66

Location—On the lateral border of the foot, antero-inferior to the 5th metatarsophalangeal joint.
Indication—Stiff neck, headache, indigestion.

U-BL-67

Location—0.1 t-sun behind and lateral to the corner of the nail of the little toe.
Indication—Painful labour, malposition of foetus.

THE PERICARDIUM MERIDIAN (Fig. 32.5)

It links 9 points of the body and obtains it's energy from the kidney meridian. It's maximum time lies between 19- 21 hours. This is the best time for a sedating treatment. Tonification is done better after this time.

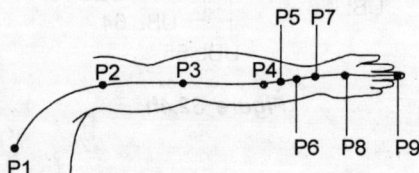

Figure 32.5: Pericardium meridian

It's starting point lies between the nipple and armpit, between the third and forth rib. It runs inside the arm and ends on the medial aspect of index finger. This meridian is not linked to any particular organ, but represents a functional cycle, which determines the peripheral circulation of the blood count and the nourishment of the Yin organ. It is linked to the bloodstream and all it's endocrine serological components and intermediary metabolic products. It also includes oxidation process.

P-1

Location—On the front of the chest in the forth intercostal space, 1 t-sun lateral to the nipple.
Indication—Palpitation, angina pectoris, thorax pain, intercostal neuralgia, enlarged lymph node.

P-2

Location—Between the long and short head of biceps brachii, 2 t-sun below the humeral end of the anterior axillary fold.
Indication—Same as P1 cough, pain at the posterior and medial side of the upper arm.

P-3

Location—Medial to biceps brachii tendon on the transverse crease of the elbow.
Indication—Palpitation, arm and forearm pain, contracture and arthritis of the elbow, tremors, chest pain.

P-4

Location—On the front of the forearm, 5 t-sun above the transverse crease of the wrist between the tendon of flexor carpi radialis and palmaris longus.
Indication—Palpitation, chest pain, pleuritis, neurasthenia, tachycardia.

P-5

Location—Anterior aspect of forearm 3 t-sun above the distal transverse wrist crease, between the flexor carpi radialis and palmaris longus tendon.
Indication—Palpitation, angina pectoris, cholera, schizophrenia, epilepsy.

P-6

Location—2 t-sun above the distal transverse wrist crease between the tendon of flexor carpi radialis and palmaris longus
Indication—Palpitation, costalgia, paralysis, polio, muscular wasting, carpel tunnel syndrome, anorexia, gastralgia, epilepsy, asthma, hiccough.

P-7

Location—Midpoint of the distal transverse wrist crease, between flexor carpi radialis and palmaris longus tendon.

Indication—Fear, insomnia, herpes, neuralgia, wristpain, intercostal neuralgia, mental disturbance, paralysis, carpal tunnel syndrome.

P-8

Location—Middle of the palm. Flex the fingers at metacarpophalangeal and interphalangeal joints so they touch the carpal part of the palm. The point between the tip of the middle and ring finger, closer to 3rd metacarpal bone.
Indication—Neuralgia, carpal tunnel syndrome, chronic skin infection, polyneuropathy of hand.

P-9

Location—Midpoint of the tip of the middle finger.
Indication—Angina pectoris, all acute emergencies, shock, dizziness, fear, hypotonia.

TRIPLE WARMER MERIDIAN (Fig. 32.6)

This meridian is a Yang meridian. It has 23 points and receives it's energy from the pericardium. It's maximum time lies between 21 to 23 hours. This is the best time for sedating treatment. It's starting point lies above the nail of the ring finger. It runs up the dorsal side of the arm across the shoulder to the clavicle, rise from here to the temple bone, circles the ear, goes down to the lower jaw bone, and ends at the outer corner of the eyes.

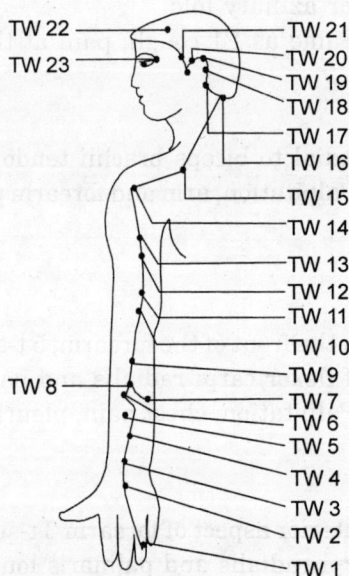

It consists of three sections

- *The lower warmer*—Which affects the urogenital system, sexual potency, and the chemical state of the whole organism.
- *The central warmer*—Which regulates the function of digestion and indigestion.
- The upper warmer-which controls respiration.

Figure 32.6: Triple warmer meridian

These three warmers represent a controlling functional cycle, which by virtue of it's opposing actions, counter balances the pericardium function.

TW-1

Location—0.1 t-sun proximal to the medial corner of the nail of the ring finger.
Indication—Headache, all acute emergencies, hyperpyrexia.

TW-2

Location—0.5 t-sun above the margin of the 4th web.
Indication—Hand pain, spastic fingers, headache.

TW-3

Location—Dorsum of the hand in the 4th intermetacarpal space in a hollow proximal to the metacarpo phalangeal joint.
Indication—Rheumatic pain of the hand, headache, deafness, vertigo, polyneuropathy.

TW-4

Location—On the dorsal aspect of the wrist crease medial to extensor digitorum Tendon.
Indication—Wrist drop, wrist arthritis.

TW–5

Location—On the dorsal aspect of the forearm, 2t-sun proximal to the dorsal transverse wrist crease between the two bones of the forearm.
Indication—Distortions, sexual weakness, pain and paralysis of upper limb, wrist drop, neck pain, deafness, arthritis of the small joint of hand and fingers, fever, migraine.

TW-6

Location—1 t-sun above TW-5.
Indication—Paralysis of upper limb.

TW-7

Location—¾ t-sun lateral to TW-6.
Indication—Pain and paralysis of upper limb, epilepsy.

TW-8

Location—2 t-sun proximal to TW-5 midway between radius and ulna.
Indication—Paralysis and pain of upper limb, deafness, intercostal neuralgia.

TW-9

Location—5 t-sun below the tip of the olecranon, between the two bones of the forearm.
Indication—Toothache, paralysis and pain of upper limb.

TW-10

Location—On the back of the elbow, 1 t-sun proximal to the tip of the olecranon process.
Indication—Hemiplegia, shoulder and arm pain, elbow joint stiffness.

TW-11

Location—1 t-sun proximal to TW-10. On the posterior side of the upper arm.
Indication—Periarthritis of shoulder.

TW-12

Location—On the posterior side of the arm 6 t-sun above olecranon.
Indication—Arm pain.

TW-13

Location—3 t-sun below TW-14. On the posterior side of the arm.
Indication—Shoulder and scapular joint pain.

TW-14

Location—It lies between the acromion and greater tubersity of the humerus, when arm is adducted.
Indication—Paralysis of upper limb, pain, periarthritis and frozen shoulder.

TW-15

Location—Midway between the tip of the acromion and center point of the intervertebral space. between C-7 and T-1.
Indication—Paralysis and pain of upper limb.

TW-16

Location—Below and behind the tip of the mastoid process, at the level of the angle of the mandible.
Indication—Stiffness of the neck, deafness.

TW-17

Location—Behind the lobule of the ear in the depression between the mastoid process and the angle of the mandible.
Indication—Facial nerve paralysis, trigeminal neuralgia, deafness.

TW-18

Location—Center of mastoid process.
Indication—Facial nerve paralysis, deafness, tinnitis.

TW-19

Location—1 t-sun above TW-18.
Indication—Deafness, otitismedia, mastoiditis.

TW-20

Location—On the natural hairline above the apex auriculae.
Indication—Toothache, otitismedia, deafness.

TW-21

Location—In the depression in front of the superior notch of the tragus when the mouth is open.
Indication—Vertigo, deafness, arthritis of temporomandibular joint.

TW-22

Location—At the level with the superior margin of the root of the auricle along, superficial temporal artery.
Indication—Facial nerve paralysis, headache.

TW-23

Location—Lateral end of the eyebrow.
Indication—Migraine, frontal sinusitis, frontal headache.

THE GALL BLADDER MERIDIAN (Figs 32.7a to c)

The gall bladder meridian is a Yang meridian. It obtains it's energy from the triple warmer meridian. Its maximum time lies between 23 to 1 hr. This is the best time for sedating treatment. Tonification is better after this time. It runs in a centrifugal direction and begins at the outer corner of the eye.

It runs across the temples and occipital zone to the central part of the trapezius, passes the shoulder joint to the top of the pelvis and along the outside of the leg to the tip of the 4th toe.

GB-1

Location—0.5 t-sun lateral to the lateral canthus of the eye.
Indication—Headache, facial paralysis, trigeminal neuralgia.

GB-2

Location—Depression in front of the inferior notch of the tragus or on the posterior margin of the condyloid process of the mandible.
Indication—Trigeminal neuralgia, upper toothache, tempromandibular joint arthritis, facial paralysis.

GB-3

Location—Anterior to the ear, the upper border of the zygomatic arch vertically above ST-7.
Indication—Facial paralysis, deafness.

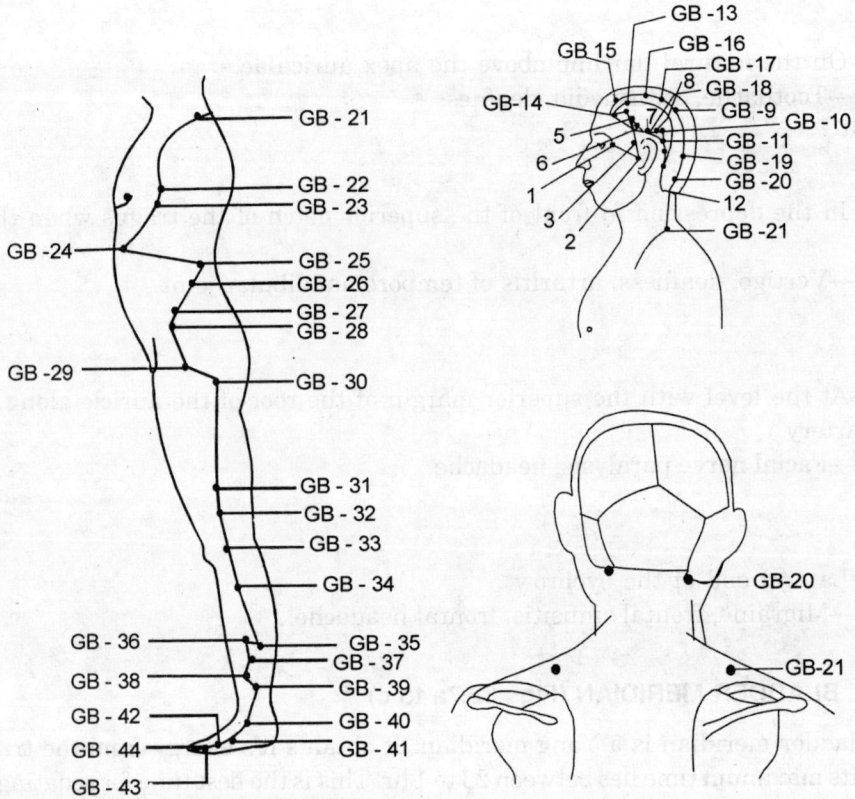

Figures 32.7a to c: Gallbladder meridian

GB-4

Location—1t-sun below on the temple.
Indication—Facial paralysis, migraine.

GB-5

Location—As above on GB-4 to GB–7 line.
Indication—Toothache, migraine.

GB-6

Location—As above on GB-4 to GB-7 line.
Indication—Same as GB-5.

GB-7

Location—Crossing point of GB-4 to GB-7 line.
Indication—Headache, stiffness of neck.

GB-8

Location—Directly above the apex of auricle, 1.5 t-sun above the natural hair line. To mark the apex auricle should be folded upon itself vertically.
Indication—Headache, vertigo, migraine.

GB-9

Location—0.5 t-sun behind GB-8, 2 t-sun, above the natural hair line.
Indication—Headache, gingivitis.

GB-10

Location—Behind the ear, 1 t-sun below GB-9 on the posterosuperior part of the mastoid process
Indication—Deafness, tonsillitis.

GB-11

Location—Midway between GB-10 and GB-12.
Indication—Eye pain, headache.

GB-12

Location—In the hallow made by bending the neck behind and below the mastoid process.
Indication—Bell's palsy, toothache.

GB-13

Location—Vertically above the outer canthus of the eye, 0.5 t-sun above the natural hairline.
Indication—Cervical spondylosis, stiffneck, facial paralysis.

GB-14

Location—On the forehead 1 t-sun vertically above the midpoint of the eyebrow.
Indication—Bell's palsy, frontal sinusitis, trigeminal neuralgia.

GB-15

Location—0.5 t-sun inside the hairline vertically above the pupil. Patient is asked to look straight ahead while locating the point.
Indication—Epilepsy, diseases of eye.

GB-16

Location—1 t-sun above GB-15.
Indication—Edema, eye diseases.

GB-17

Location—1 t-sun behind and 1t-sun above GB-15.
Indication—Toothache, headache.

GB-18

Location—1t-sun above, 1.5 t-sun behind GB-15.
Indication—Headache, blocked nose.

GB-19

Location—1.5 t-sun above GB-20 lateral to the external occipital protuberance
Indication—Cervical spondylosis, bronchial asthma.

GB-20

Location—At the apex of posterior triangle of the neck, in the hallow directly below and between the external occipital protuberance and the mastoid process. It lies between the insertion of the trapezius and sternocleidomastoid.
Indication—Headache, stiff neck., hypertension, vertigo, cervical spondylosis.

GB-21

Location—It is situated midway between GV-14 and acromion.
Indication—Backache, cervical spondylosis, frozen shoulder, motor disorders of upper limb functional uterine bleeding, stiff neck.

GB-22

Location—3 t-sun below the mid axillary fold.
Indication—Intercostal neuralgia, pleuritis.

GB-23

Location—On the chest in the 4th intercostal space 1 t-sun anterior to GB-22.
Indication—Heartburn, bronchial asthma, hyperacidity, gallcolic, flatulance.

GB-24

Location—In the 7th intercostal space directly below the nipple.
Indication—Lactation problem, epigastric pain, migraine.

GB-25

Location—On the abdominal wall at the lower border of the free end of the 12th rib.
Indication—Hepatic disorder, fever, intercostal neuralgia, gallcolic.

GB-26

Location—On the abdominal wall, midway between the free ends of the 11th and 12th ribs at the level of umbilicus.
Indication—Lumbago, intercostal neuralgia, dysmenorrhoea, menorrhagia, cystitis.

GB-27

Location—In the front of the anterior superior iliac spine at the level with CV-4.
Indication—Lower abdominal pain, endometriosis

GB-28

Location—0.5 t-sun below anterior to GB-27.
Indication—Lower abdominal pain, dysmenorrhoea, constipation.

GB-29

Location—Midway between the highest point of the greater trochanter of the femur and the anterior superior iliac spine.
Indication—Lumbago, lowerabdominal pain, hip joint arthritis.

GB-30

Location—At the junction of the outer 1/3 and the middle 2/3 of a line drawn between the highest point of the greater trochanter and sacral hiatus.

GB-31

Location—7 t-sun above the outer end of the transverse popliteal crease on the lateral aspect of the thigh.
Indication—Polio, lower limb paralysis, sciatica, lumbago.

GB-32

Location—2 t-sun below the GB-31.
Indication—Sciatica, hemiplegia, slipped disc.

GB-33

Location—3t-sun vertically above GB-34 on the outer aspect of the knee.
Indication—Knee pain, lower limb pain and paralysis.

GB-34

Location—On the antero-lateral aspect of the leg in the depression in front and below the head of the fibula.

Indication—Hemiplegia, lumbago, vertigo, knee pain, muscle pain, polio, myopathies, muscular dystrophies, foot drop, dizziness.

GB-35

Location—On the anterior border of fibula 7 t-sun above the tip of the lateral malleolus.
Indication—Asthma, sciatica.

GB-36

Location—1 t-sun behind GB-35.
Indication—Leg cramp, stiff neck, sciatica.

GB-37

Location—2 t-sun below GB-35 in front of the fibula.
Indication—Sciatica pain in the lateral aspect of the leg, headache.

GB-38

Location—3 t-sun below GB-35 in front of the fibula.
Indication—Knee pain, and arthritis, lumbago.

GB-39

Location—3 t-sun above the lateral malleolus.
Indication—Paralysis, poliomyelitis, cervical spondylosis.

GB-40

Location—In the depression anterior and inferior to the lateral malleolus.
Indication—Costalgia, sciatica, footdrop, ankle pain and arthritis, hip pain, chronic ulcer of ankle.

GB-41

Location—In the depression anterior to the 4th intercostal joint.
Indication—Metatarsalgia, costalgia.

GB-42

Location—4th intermetatarsal space 0.5 t-sun distal to GB-41.
Indication—Axilla pain, tinnitus.

GB-43

Location—0.5 t-sun proximal to the margin of the 4th web.
Indication—Dizziness, intercostal neuralgia.

GB-44

Location—On the lateral side of the tip of the 4th toe. 0.1 t-sun proximal to the corner of the nail.
Indication—Asthma, pleuritis.

THE LIVER MERIDIAN (Fig. 32.8)

The liver meridian is a Yin meridian. It obtains it's energy from triple warmer. This channel starts from the lateral aspect of the greater toe, ascends to the dorsum of foot till medial malleolus. Further ascends to medial aspect of knee and thigh up to lower abdomen. From the level of symphysis pubis it goes up to 11rib and ends in the 6th intercostal space below the nipple.

LIV-1

Location—On the outer side of the dorsum of the terminal phalanx of the big toe, midway between the interphalangeal joint and the lateral corner of the nail.
Indication—Prolapse uterus, menorrhagia, hernia, colic.

LIV-2

Location—On the dorsum of the foot.0.5 t-sun proximal to the margin of the web between the big toe and the second toe.
Indication—Intercostal neuralgia, insomnia, headache, infantile convulsion.

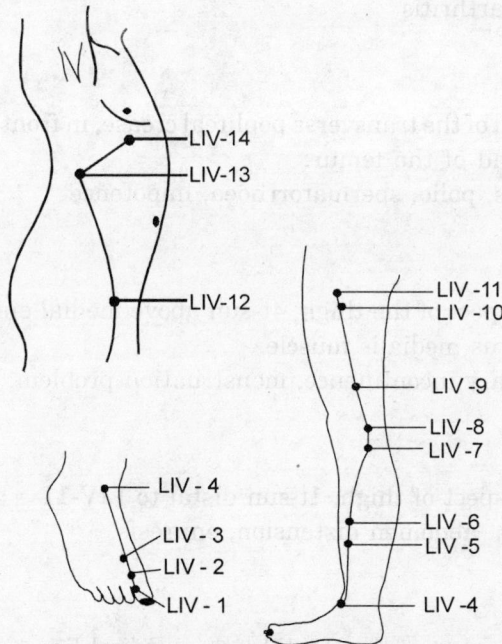

Figure 32.8: Liver meridian

LIV-3

Location—On the dorsum of the foot, in the first intermetatarsal space 2t-sun proximal to the margin of the web.
Indication—Hypertension, headache, eye disorder.

LIV-4

Location—On the ankle 1 t-sun anterior to the medial mallolus in between the tendons of the extensor hallusis longus and tibialis anterior.

LIV-5

Location—On the medial aspect of the leg, along the posterior border of the tibia.5 t-sun above the tip of the medial malleolus
Indication—Pain in lower stomach, menstruation disturbances, impotance, muscular pain.

LIV-6

Location—2 t-sun above LIV-5 on the posterior border of the tibia.
Indication—Lower limb joint pain, menorrhagia, gall bladder, and liver disorder.

LIV-7

Location—1t-sun behind sp-9 on the posterio-inferior aspect of the medial condyle of the tibia.
Indication—Knee pain and arthritis

LIV-8

Location—On the medial end of the transverse popliteal crease, in front of the semimembrenous muscle behind the lower end of the femur.
Indication—Prolapse uterus, polio, spermatorrhoea, impotence.

LIV-9

Location—On the medial aspect of the thigh, 4t-sun above medial epicondyle of the femur in between Sartorius and vastus medialis muscle.
Indication—Lumbago, urinary incontinence, menstruation problem, lower abdominal pain.

LIV-10

Location—On the medial aspect of thigh, 1t-sun distal to LIV-11
Indication—Urine retention, abdomen distension, enuresis.

LIV-11

Location—On the anterior aspect of the thigh below inguinal ligament, 1 t-sun distal to the lateral wall of the femoral artery.
Indication—Lumbago, Paraplegia, leg pain, pain, femoral neuralgia, irregular menstruation.

LIV-12

Location—2.5 t-sun lateral from the center of the symphysis pubis, in the inferio-lateral part of the pubic tubercle.
Indication—Prolapse uterus, lower abdominal pain, penis pain, pelvic cellulitis.

LIV-13

Location—On the tip of the free end of the 11th rib.
Indication—Abdominal distension, flatulence, subcostal pain, liver and spleen disorders.

LIV-14

Location—On the front of the chest directly below the nipple, on the 6th inter costal space.
Indication—Chest pain, bronchial asthma, neuralgia, pleurisy, hepatitis.

THE LUNG MERIDIAN (Figs 32.9a and b)

The lung meridian is a Yin meridian. It has 11 points and obtains its energy from the large intestine. It runs in a centrifugal direction. It's starting point ins near the armpit between the 2nd and 3rd rib and runs inside the upper and lower arms and ends on the inside of the thumb.

L-1

Location—6-t-sun lateral to the mid-line in 1st intercostal space, on the front of the chest near the coracoid process.
Indication—Haemoptysis, chest pain, asthma, bronchitis, dyspnoea, cough.

L-2

Location—In the infraclavicular fossa 6t-sun lateral to the mid-line.
Indication—Asthma, periarthritis of shoulder.

L-3

Location—3 t-sun below the axilla at the internal side of the biceps.
Indication—Chest pain, cough, asthma, dyspnoea.

L-4

Location—1 t-sun below L-3 on the medial aspect of the upper arm, antero-lateral to the humerus.
Indication—Chest pain, cough, dyspnoea.

L-5

Location—On the front of the elbow, in the depression lateral to the tendon of biceps brachii, slightly flexed elbow makes the tendon prominent, which makes easier to locate the point.

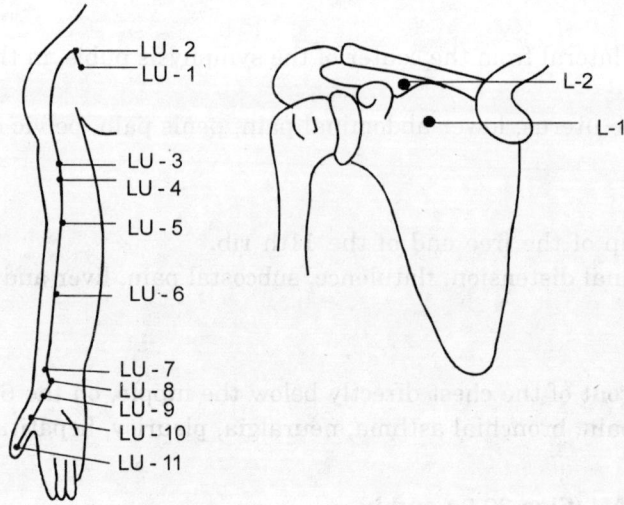

Figures 32.9a and b: The lung meridian

Indication—Asthma, coughs, sore throat, painful arm, neuropathies of upper limb, paralysis of upper limb, psoriasis, dermatitis.

L-6. (Fig. 32.9c)

Location—On the radial side of the forearm 7t-sun proximal to the distal wrist crease (L-9)

Indication—Asthmatic bronchitis, dyspnoea, cough, haemoptysis.

L-7

Location—1.5 t-sun proximal to the distal wrist crease, on the outer aspect of the forearm.

Indication—Wrist drop, wrist arthritis, bell's palsy, cervical spondylosis, bronchitis, asthma, headache, paralysis of upper limb, parkinsonism.

L-8

Location—1 t-sun proximal to distal wrist crease on the medial side of the radial styloid process lateral to radial artery.

Indication—Cough, asthma, wrist and hand pain, dyspnoea.

L-9

Location—On the lateral end of the distal transverse wrist crease, lateral to the radial artery.

Indication—Cough, asthma, bronchitis, raynaud's disease, varicose ulcer and varicose vein, burger's disease, myoneuropathies of the upper limb, carpel tunnel syndrome, wrist and hand pain, backache, shoulder pain.

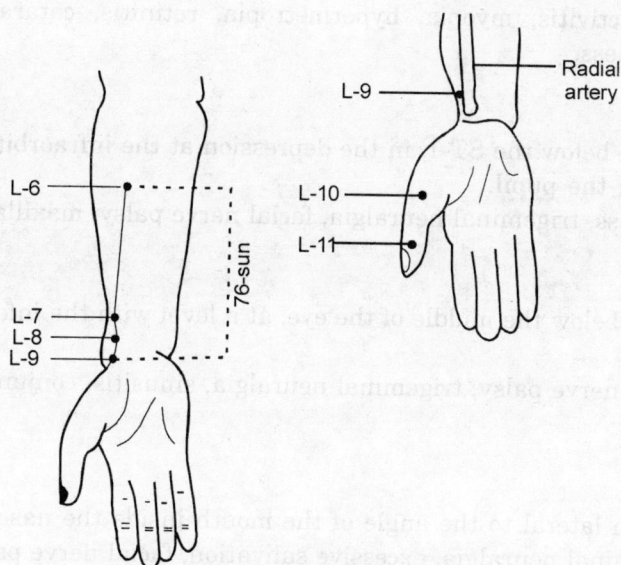

Figure 32.9c

L-10

Location—On the thenar eminence of the palm, over middle of the first metacarpal. Bone, at the junction of the two colors of the skin.

Indication—Carpel tunnel syndrome, hand pain, polyneuropathy, paresthesia of hand, cough, asthma, haemoptysis.

L-11

Location—On the lateral side of the thumb 0.1 t-sun proximal to the corner of the nail.

Indication—Shock, cardiac arrest, coma, respiratory failure, apoplexy, cramps headache, angina, and epilepsy.

THE STOMACH MERIDIAN (Figs 32.10a and b)

The stomach meridian is a Yang meridian. It has 45 points, and receives it's energy from the colon meridian. The stomach meridian runs in a centrifugal direction. It begins at the naso labial fold, then runs along the lower jawbone, to the vicinity of the temples, and then returns to the lower jaw bone, where it runs via the clavicle and nipple and passes navel to the hip, then along the front side of the thigh and lower leg till it ends on the top section of the second toe.

ST-1

Location—Below the eye on the midpoint of the infraorbital ridge.

Indication—Conjunctivitis, myopia, hypermetropia, retinitis, cataracts, night blindness, astigmatism, blindness.

ST-2

Location—0.7 t-sun below the ST-1, in the depression at the infraorbital foramen, vertically below the center of the pupil.
Indication—Deafness, trigeminal neuralgia, facial nerve palsy, maxillary sinusitis.

ST-3

Location—Directly below the middle of the eye, at a level with the inferior border of the ala-nasi.
Indication—Facial nerve palsy, trigeminal neuralgia, sinusitis, conjunctivitis, toothache, stuttering.

ST-4

Location—0.4 t-sun lateral to the angle of the mouth inside the nasolabial sulcus.
Indication—Trigeminal neuralgia, excessive salivation, facial nerve palsy, aphasia.

ST-5

Location—In front of the angle of the mandible on the antero-inferior border of the masseter muscle behind the facial artery. It is helpful to palpate the artery on the mandible to locate the point.
Indication—Paralysis, toothache, trigeminal neuralgia.

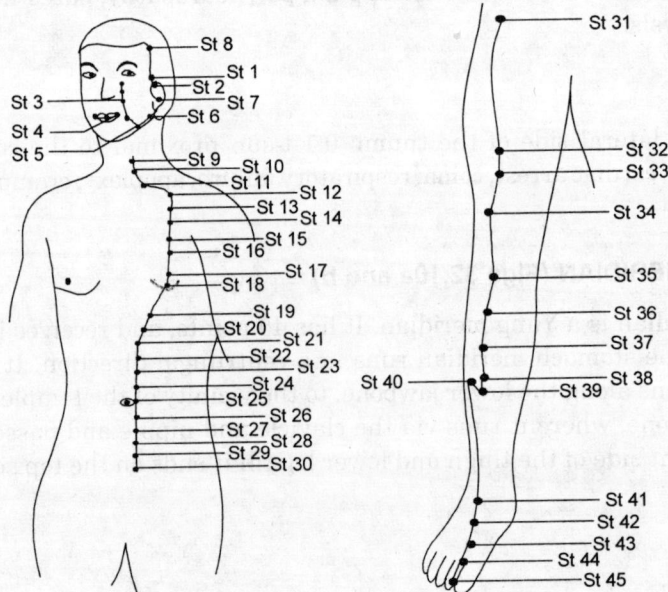

Figures 32.10a and b: The stomach meridian

ST-6

Location—Over the masseteri muscle anterior to the angle of the mandible for better location ask the patient to clench the teeth.
Indication—Toothache, facial nerve palsy, myopia, swollen jaw skin disorder of mouth.

ST-7

Location—In the center of the depression of the lower margin of the zygomatic arch, anterior to temporomandibular joint.
Indication—Toothache, facial nerve palsy, dislocation of temporo mandibular joint, deafness, inflammation of the mandible, trigeminal neuralgia.

ST-8

Location—At the angle of the forehead 0.5 t-sun inside the natural anterior hairline.
Indication—Migraine, eyepain, headache, frontal sinusitis, giddiness.

ST-9

Location—By the side of the laryngeal prominence behind common carotid artery.
Indication—Sore throat, aphasia, asthma, hypertension, dysarthria, vomiting, tonsillitis, dyspnoea.

ST-10

Location—On the front of the sternocleido mastoidmuscle, midway between ST-9 and ST-11.
Indication—Asthma, tracheitis, sore throat.

ST-11

Location—On the superior border of the medial end of the clavicle, in between the two heads of the sternocleidomastoid muscle directly below ST-9.
Indication—Stiffneck, neck pain, cough, chest pain.

ST-12

Location—In the middle of the supraclavicular fossa vertically above the nipple.
Indication—Asthma, intercostal neuralgia, insomnia, angina, bronchitis, dyspnoea.

ST-13

Location—Mid point of the infraclavicular region.
Indication—Chest pain, asthma, bronchitis, dyspnoea.

ST-14

Location—Under the first rib on the mamillary line.
Indication—Bronchitis, chest pain, asthma.

ST-15

Location—Under the 2nd rib on the mamillary line.
Indication—Asthma, gastritis, chest abscess, bronchitis.

ST-16

Location—Under the 3rd rib on the mamillary line.
Indication—Diarrhoea, asthma, cough, ribpain, bronchitis.

ST-17

Location—Center of the nipple.
Indication—Asthma, angina, cough, diarrhoea.

ST-18

Location—Mid clavicular line, in 5th intercostal space, below the nipple.
Indication—Pain and heaviness of chest, intercostal neuralgia, cough, breast infection, placenta retention mammillitis.

ST-19

Location—6 t-sun above the umbilicus and 2 t-sun lateral to the midline.
Indication—Dry mouth, cough, stomach ulcer, gastritis, intercostal neuralgia, abdominal pain.

ST-20

Location—5 t-sun above the umbilicus and 2 t-sun lateral to the midline.
Indication—Stomach pain, nausea, epigastric pain.

ST-21

Location—4 t-sun above the umbilicus and 2 t-sun lateral to the midline.
Indication—Spastic colon, gall bladder colic, gastroneurosis, umbilical and incisional hernia.

ST-22

Location—3 t-sun above the umbilicus and 2 t-sun lateral to the midline.
Indication—Anorexia, diarrhoea, oedema, abdominal pain, fever, incontinence.

ST-23

Location—2t-sun above the umbilicus and 2t-sun lateral to the midline.
Indication—Acute gastritis, bowel colic, abdominal pain.

ST-24

Location—1 t-sun above the umbilicus and 2 t-sun lateral to the midline.
Indication—Nausea, epigastric pain, gastralgia.

ST-25

Location—2 t-sun lateral to umbilicus over rectus abdominis muscle.
Indication—All chemical stomach disorders, such as sickness, stomach ache, constipation, diarrhoea, bowelcramp, menstruation disorders, sterility, cholera, oedema, vomiting, chorea.

ST-26

Location—1 t-sun below and 2 t-sun lateral to midline.
Indication—Depression, dysentery, vomiting, paralysis of abdominal muscle, acute and chronic gastroenteritis.

ST-27

Location—2 t-sun below ST-25.
Indication—Oedema, nephritis insomnia, gastralgia, gastric, intestinal colic.

ST-28

Location—3 t-sun below ST-25 2 t-sun lateral to midline.
Indication—Urine retention, cystitis, nephritis, oedema.

ST-29

Location—4 t-sun below ST-25 and 2 t-sun lateral to midline.
Indication—Amenorrhoea, irregular menstruation, urogenital disorders, leucorrhoea, prolapse uterus.

ST-30

Location—5 t-sun below ST-25 and 2 t-sun lateral to midline in the inguinal region.
Indication—Lower bowel disorders, hernia, anorexia, dysmenorrhoea, amenorrhoea, frigidity, impotence.

ST-31

Location—In the line of the lower border of the pubic symphysis, directly below the anterior superior iliac spine.
Indication—Paraplegia, hemiplegia, polio, lumbago, gonorrhoea, hip pain and stiffness of joint, lower abdominal pain.

ST-32

Location—6 t-sun above the upper margin of the patella between rectus femoris and vastus lateralis.
Indication—Arthritis of knee, muscle weakness of lower limb, asthma, wasting of quadriceps, gonorrhoea.

ST-33

Location—3 t-sun above the upper and outer margin of the patella
Indication—Knee pain, paralysis of lower limb diabetes, foot cramps, oedema of leg.

ST-34

Location—In a depression on the front of thigh 2t-sun above the upper and outer edge of petella, vertically above the lateral foramen of patella.
Indication—Diarrhoea, cold leg, knee joint pain, epigastric pain, facial neuralgia.

ST-35

Location—Below the patella, lateral to ligamentum patella. It is best to locate in slightly flexed knee.
Indication—Arthritis and pain of knee joint, polio, weakness of leg muscle, oedema of knee.

ST-36

Location—One finger breadth lateral to the lower border of the tibial tuberosity or 3 t-sun below ST-35.
Indication—Epilepsy, fatigue, weakness, polio, polyneuropathy, gastralgia, anorexia, vomiting, gastritis, constipation, diabetes, hypertension, varicose vein, palpitation, nervousness.

ST-37

Location—6 t-sun below ST-35 one finger breadth lateral to the anterior border of the tibia on the lateral aspect of the leg.
Indication—Chronic appendicitis, gastritis, colitis, hemiplegia, abdominal pain.

ST-38

Location—5 t-sun below ST-36.
Indication—Knee infection, calf muscle pain and cramp, tonsillitis, knee arthritis, paralysis of lower limb, periarthritis, epigastric pain.

ST-39

Location—3 t-sun below ST-36.
Indication—Brain anemia, dry skin, tonsillitis, epigastric pain, paralysis of lower limb.

ST-40

Location—5 t-sun below ST-36 and 2 finger breadth lateral to the anterior border of the tibia.
Indication—Hemiplegia, paralysis of lower limb, cough, oedema, bronchial asthma.

ST-41

Location—On the dorsum of the foot at the midpoint of the transverse crease of ankle.
Indication—Oedema of face, swelling and pain of lower limb, foot drop, hemiplegia, varicose vein, arthritis and pain of ankle.

ST-42

Location—On the highest spot of the dorsum of the foot.1.5 t-sun distal to the ST-41 by the side of dorsal is pedis artery.
Indication—Palpitation, toothache, paralysis of lower limb, epilepsy.

ST-43

Location—Between the 2nd and 3rd metatarsal bone, on the dorsum of the foot.
Indication—Anorexia, paraplegia, stomach ulcer, oedema of face, foot oedema, polyneuropathy, toothache, abdominal pain.

ST-44

Location—On the dorsal aspect of the foot 0.5 t-sun proximal to the web space between the second and third toes.
Indication—Stomach ache, dyspepsia, anorexia, ankle arthritis, paralysis of lower limb, polyneuropathy, headache, toothache.

ST-45

Location—0.1 t-sun proximal to the lateral side of the corner of the nail of the 2nd toe.
Indication—Dyspepsia, toothache, migraine, fainting, epilepsy, hyper pyrexia.

THE SPLEEN –PANCREAS MERIDIAN (Figs 32.11a and b)

The spleen meridian is a Yin meridian. It has 21 points and obtains it's energy from the stomach meridian. It's starting point is on the medialside of the upper section of the big toe, from there it runs along inside of the leg, reaching the navel and then passes the nipple, until it ends in the vicinity of the 2nd intercostal space.

SP-1

Location—On the medial side of the great toe 0.1 t-sun proximal to the medial corner of the nail.
Indication—Insomania, fear, asthma, hyperacidity, abdominal distension, menstrual disorders.

SP-2

Location—On the medial side of the big toe, antero-inferior to the 1st metatarsophalangeal joint.
Indication—Diabetes, rheumatic pain, high fever, epigastric pain, abdominal distension.

SP-3

Location—On the inner aspect of the foot postero inferior to the head of the 1st metatarsal bone at the junction of the two colors of skin.
Indication—Headache, excitement, swollen thorax, hyperacidity, nausea, gastralgia, flatulence, dysentry, constipation.

SP-4

Location—On the inner aspect of the foot in the proximal end of the 1st metatarsal bone at the junction of the two colours of the skin.
Indication—Swollen stomach, dysmenorrhoea, diarrhoea, oedema, epigastric pain, gastralgia, dyspepsia.

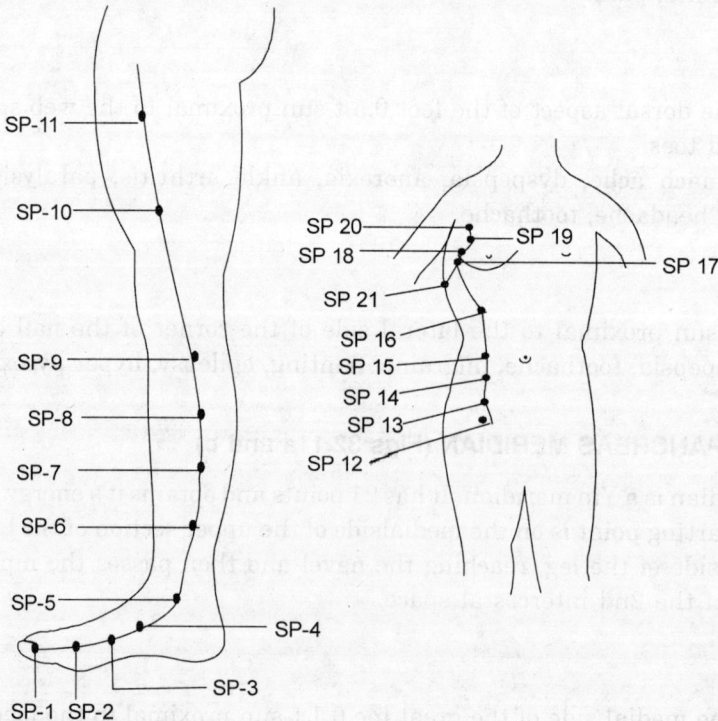

Figures 32.11a and b: The spleen meridian

SP-5

Location—At the crossing of the two lines drawn along the anterior and inferior borders of the medial malleolus.
Indication—Sedating point, stomachache, gastritis, headache, arthritis, ankle pain, planter fascitis.

SP-6

Location—3 t-sun proximal to the tip of medial malleolus just behind the medial border and posterior surface of the tibia.
Indication—Nervous depression, vertigo, diarrhoea, abdominal distension, lower abdominal pain. Dysmenorrhoea, Leucorrhoea, Spermatorrhoea, diseases of genito—urinary organ, dysuria, urine retention, psoriasis, eczema hemiplegia, diabetes, foot drop, myopathies, fatigue, polyneuropathy, varicose vein, low blood pressure, liver and kidney disorders.

SP-7

Location—6 t-sun above the apex of the medial malleolus behind the tibia.
Indication—Indigestion, flatulence, hyperperistalsis, leg and knee numbness.

SP-8

Location—3 t-sun below SP-9.
Indication—Stiff neck, menorrhagia, neuralgia, lumbago, abdominal distension.

SP-9

Location—In the groove of the lower border of the medial condyle of the tibia in a level with the lower border of the tibia tuberosity.
Indication—Stomach cramp, incontinence, dysuria, dysentery, oedema, menstrual disturbances.

SP-10

Location—2 t-sun proximal to the superior border of the patella on the antero medial aspect of the thigh.
Indication—Disorders of the knee joint, psoriasis, pneumonitis, genito-urinary diseases, orchitis, exzema, menstrual disturbances.

SP-11

Location—8 t-sun above the antero-medial border of patella, medial to the sartorius muscle.
Indication—Incontinence, enuresis, dysria, inguinal lymphadenitis.

SP-12

Location—3.5 t-sun lateral to the mid point of the upper border of the symphysis pubis, lateral to the femoral artery.
Indication—Swollen stomach, breast infection, stomach cramp, hernia, blood in urine.

SP-13

Location—4 t-sun lateral to the midline of the anterior abdominal wall, 0.7 t-sun above SP-12.
Indication—Bowel cramps, hernia, stomach ache, constipation, appendicitis.

SP-14

Location—4 t-sun lateral to the midline and 1.5 t-sun below the umbilicus.
Indication—Hernia, dyspnoe, diarrhoea, paraumbilical pain.

SP-15

Location—Vertically below the nipple 4 t-sun lateral to the umbilicus.
Indication—Epilepsy, influenza, diarrhoea, constipation, epigastric pain, paralytic ileus.

SP-16

Location—3 t-sun above SP-15, 4 t-sun lateral to midline.
Indication—Constipation, bowel parasites, dyspepsia, abdominal pain, dysentery.

SP-17

Location—5th intercostals space, 6 t-sun lateral to the midline.
Indication—Congestion of lungs, chest and subcostal pain, heaviness in chest.

SP-18

Location—4th intercostals space 6 t-sun lateral to the midline.
Indication—Bronchitis, stomach ulcer, mastitis, lactational disorders, cough, chest pain intercostals neuralgia.

SP-19

Location—3rd intercostals space, 6 t-sun lateral to midline.
Indication—Same as SP-18

SP-20

Location—2nd intercostals space, 6 t-sun lateral to the midline.
Indication—Dyspnoe, cough, costal and subcostal pain.

SP-21

Location—6th intercostals space in the mid axillary line.
Indication—Dyspnoea, costal pain, bodyache. This is the luo point for spleen.

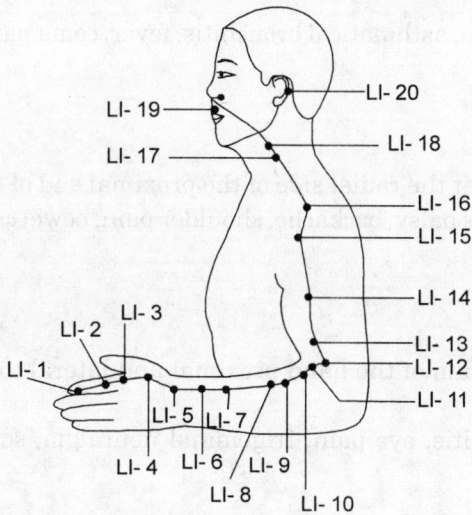

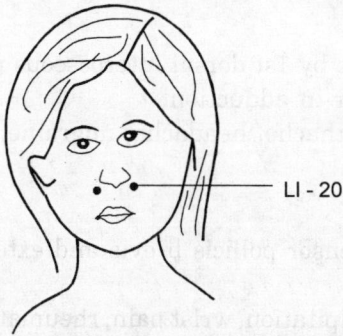

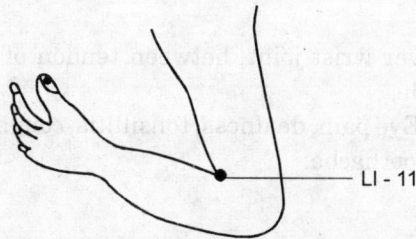

Figures 32.12a to c: The large intestine meridian

THE LARGE INTESTINE MERIDIAN (Figs 32.12a to c)

The large intestine meridian is a yang meridian, which receives its energy from the lung meridian. It runs in a centripetal direction.

The starts from the tip of the radial side of the index finger near the root of the nail. It runs from there along the outer side of the top section of index finger, continues along the outer ventral side of the arm to the clavicle, through more in the vicinity of the breast bone. It runs via the lower jawbone and the corner of the mouth to the opposite nasolabial fold where it ends.

LI-1

Location—0.1 t-sun proximal to the corner of the nail of the index finger on the radial side.

Indication—Sinusitis, deafness, asthma, asthmatical bronchitis, fever, coma paraesthesia of the finger.

LI-2

Location—On the dorsum of the hand at the radial side of the proximal end of the index finger.
Indication—Toothache, laryngitis, bell's palsy, backache, shoulder pain, bowel cramp, diarrhoea, stomach ache.

LI-3

Location—In a depression on the dorsum of the hand proximal and lateral to the head of the second metacarpal bone.
Indication—Angina, bowel cramp, colitis, eye pain, trigeminal neuralgia, sore throat, lower toothache.

LI-4

Location—On the highest point of the bulging made by 1st dorsal interosseous muscle when the thumb and index finger are held close together in adduction.
Indication— Bell's Palsy, trigeminal neuralgia, toothache, headache, migraine, sore throat.

LI-5

Location—Over wrist joint, between tendon of extensor pollicis brevis and extensor pollicis longus muscle.
Indication—Eye pain, deafness, tonsillitis, cough, palpitation, wrist pain, rheumatoid arthritis, wrist drop, toothache.

LI-6

Location—On the radial side of the back of the wrist 3 t-sun above LI-5
Indication—Facial Palsy, pain and swelling in forearm, skin diseases, fever, oedema.

LI-7

Location—5 t-sun above LI-5 on a line joining LI-5 and LI-11
Indication—Headache, nausea, shoulder pain and stiffness, hepatitis, gastro intestinal disorders parotitis.

LI-8

Location—4 t-sun distal to LI-11
Indication—Headache, dry lips, stomachache, indigestion, arm and elbow neuralgia, mastitis.

LI-9

Location—3 t-sun distal to L-11
Indication—Paralysis and paraesthesia of upper limb, shoulder pain, back pain, paresis, headache, gonorrhoea, flatulence.

LI-10

Location—2 t-sun distal to LI –11
Indication—Shoulder pain, stomach ache, diarrhoea, migraine, angina, pruritis, hemiplegia, elbow arthritis.

LI-11

Location—Semi flex elbow on the lateral end of the elbow crease.
Indication—Hypertension, epicondilytis, shoulder pain, back ache, skin diseases paralysis of upper limb.

LI-12

Location—1 t-sun above LI-11
Indication—Brachialgie, stiffness, pain and contracture of elbow, tennis elbow myositis ossification.

LI-13

Location—3 t-sun above LI-11
Indication—Paralysis of arm and leg, elbow pain and arthritis of upper limb, pneumonia.

LI-14

Location—7 t-sun proximal to the LI-11 at the level of insertion of deltoid, on the line joining LI-11 and LI-15.
Indication—Frozen shoulder, hemiplegia, headache, eye disease.

LI-15

Location—On the depression at antero-inferior border of acromioclavicular joint when the arm is adducted.
Indication—Frozen shoulder, paralysis of upper limb, painful are syndrome, sprain of shoulder, hypertension, dry skin.

LI-16

Location—At the depression between the acromial end of the clavicle and the upper part of the spine of the scapula
Indication—Brachialgia, convulsion, frozen shoulder, backache.

LI-17

Location—1 t-sun below LI-18 at the posterior border of sternocleidomastoid.
Indication—Tuberculosis of cervical lymphnode, pharyngitis.

LI-18

Location—On the neck 3 t-sun lateral to the middle of the laryngeal prominence, between the two heads of the sterno-cleido-mastoid.
Indication—Lung diseases, cough, sore throat, enlarged thyroid, aphasia.

LI-19

Location—0.5 t-sun by the side of the GV—26 below the lateral margin of the nostril.
Indication—Hayfever, blocked nose, sinusitis, facial palsy, trigeminal neuralgia, smoking addiction.

LI-20

Location—Mid point on the line drawn horizontally from the highest point of the ala-nasi towards naso-labial groove on the opposite side.
Indication—Sinusitis, trigeminal neuralgia, upper toothache, facial paralysis, maxillary sinusitis, cold.

chapter thirty-three

Moxibustion

The dry powder of the leaf of "Artemisia valgaris" is known as "Moxa" and when the powder is used for therapy known as "Moxibustion". It is a method of treating diseases by applying heat on acupuncture points.

It is generally indicated in chronic diseases of cold or diseases caused by an excess of yin energy. Diseases like bronchial asthma, chronic bronchitis, paralysis, arthritis, moxibustion is very useful.

Moxa can be used in various way—moxa cone, moxa roll, moxa sticks, cigars. Using these treatment can be given is following ways.

Direct Moxibustion

A small moxa cone is placed directly on the treatment point.

  i. Scarring moxibustion—Moxa Cone is kept directly on the acupuncture point until skin is burnt. This results in the formation of blisters, therefore, it is not in much use, it is very effective in chronic allergies.
  ii. Non-scarring moxibustion—A cone is kept over the acupuncture point and removed as soon as a sensation of scorching with slight pain is felt. There is no blister or scar formation with this method.

Indirect Moxibustion

In this method moxa is not kept directly on the body. A medium should be kept in between the skin and moxa, which can be ginger, garlic or salt.

In this method ginger or garlic is used as a medium between moxa and skin. Slice of ginger or garlic is made moxa is kept over them and burnt. Acupuncture point is stimulated by the heat crossing the medium. This can be repeated 3 to 5 times until the desired effect is obtained.

Moxibustion is avoided in very hairy area, near the sensory organ, large blood vessels, poor circulation, ulcer and mucous membrane.

It should not be used in small children, nervous, diabetic, mentally deficient patient. Yang disorders are contraindicated.

chapter thirty-four

Therapy Index

1. Acne   -   LI–13, JM–15
2. Abscess   -   LI–4 and 11, ST–2, 3, 6
3. Allergy   -   LI–5, 14
4. Anemia   -   UB–17, 43, 42, ST–36
5. Anxiety   -   P–6, HT, SP–4
7. Facial Paralysis   -   St–6, 7
8. Urine or farces   -   UB–32, 40
   Incontinence
9. Lumbago Arthrose   -   UB–23, 25, 40
10. Thorax Arthrose   -   DM–14, 6
11. Elbow Arthrose   -   TN–5, LV–5, LI–11
12. Shoulder Arthrose   -   TW–5, 14, Si–3, 10
13. Wrist Arthrose   -   LI–4, 5, TW–3, Si–4
14. Finger Arthrose   -   LI–4, Si–3
15. Hip Arthrose   -   GB–29, 30, UB–40, 23, 25, 32, 31
16. Knee Arthrose   -   GB–30, 32, 34, 39, St–32, 36, 44
17. Asthma   -   UB–13, 17, LU–1, 2, St–12, 36
18. Bronchitis   -   Acute–LU–5, 7, LI–4,
                                 Chronic–UB–12, 13, LU–1, 2, 7,
                                 K–6, 24, 25, St–18
19. Brachialgia   -   St–38, UB–57, GB–20, 34
20. Backache   -   UB–18
21. Cholestrol   -   SP–2, 3, Li–3
22. Constipation   -   TW–6, Li–3, Si–8, St–25
23. Depression   -   St–36, UB–15, GB–34
24. Diarrhoea   -   St–25, 36, SP–4
25. Dysmenorrhea   -   UB–26, Li–3, St–4,
26. Flatulence   -   St–25, 36, SP–6
27. Gastritis   -   St–36, P –6, SP–4, UB–21
28. Haemorrhoid   -   UB–57, SP–1, P–6
29. Headache   -   St–36, LI–4, UB–60
30. Hypertension   -   UB–15, Li–3, LI–4, St–36
                                 GB–34, 39
31. Hemiplegia   -   K–6, UB–62
32. Incontinence   -   K–9, SP–6

33.	Lumbago	-	UB–23, 31, 32, 33, 40
34.	Mental Retardation	-	UB–15, 39, 62, Lou–9, K–7
35.	Migraine	-	St–1, GB–8, UB–60, SP–6
36	Polio	-	TW–5, LI–11
37.	Arm Paralysis	-	LI–4, 11, Si–6, 7
38.	Hand Paralysis	-	TW–5, 9, Si–6, P–8, UB–36
39.	Leg Paralysis	-	UB–40, 58, 60, Si–31, 33, 36
40.	Rheumatism	-	TW–5, SP–6
41.	Sinusitis	-	GB–20, co4
42.	Tachycardia	-	P–6, H–5
43.	Vertigo	-	GB–3, DM–20
44.	Menstruation Problem	-	St–36, SP–6

SECTION 6
NUTRITION

chapter thirty-five

Introduction and Definitions

Food is something we eat and which is utilised by our body to give energy. Food has been a basic part of our existence.

Food, which provides energy, building, regulation and protection of the body. While NUTRITION is the combination of processes by which we utilise food.

The process by which the body utilises food is called nutrition. The food is first consumed by us and is utilised by our body by the process of digestion, absorption, transport, storage, metabolism and elimination for the purpose of maintenance of life, growth, and normal functioning of organs and production of energy.

Nutrition is thus a sum total of all these process by which living being receives and utilise the food necessary for the maintenance of their function and growth and renewal of their component.

Nutrient includes water, proteins, fat, carbohydrates, minerals, and vitamins. Our body requires these nutrients in adequate amount to promote good health.

Nutritional status   It is the condition of health of the individual as influenced by the utilisation of the nutrients. It can be good or poor nutritional state.

Malnutrition   It is an impairment of health resulting from a deficiency, excess or imbalance of nutrients. It includes undernutrition, which refers to a deficiency of calories or one or more essential nutrients.

Overnutrition   Which is an excess of one or more nutrients and usually of calories.

Diet   Diet is whatever we eat and drink each day. Diet can be normal, which we consume everyday and it can be modified and used for ill person as a part of the whole therapy, i.e. therapeutic diet.

RECOMMENDED DIET ALLOWANCE

RDA   The RDA indicates how much of a nutrient a person needs. It is given as a daily value, but it is safe to take more or less on any particular day if the intake over several days is atleast the RDA.

chapter thirty-six

Function of Food

Food is our basic necessity. We may live without food for few days but if we don't eat for long, our working capacity goes down, we may feel weak. This indicates that the food is important for maintaining our general health and it helps us to perform various activities.

Function can be of following ways

1. Physiological function
2. Psychological function
3. Social function.

PHYSIOLOGICAL FUNCTION

- Energy giving
- Body building
- Regulation of body process

Energy Giving Function

Food is utilised in our body to give energy. The body needs energy to sustain the involuntary processes, essential for continuance of life, and for performing various physical activities.

The energy needed for body function is supplied by the oxidation of the food consumed apart from these, energy is also required for some of the involuntary process, such as blood circulation, respiration, digestion, and absorption of food, excretion of waste product. Energy value of food is measured in kilocalories.

A KILO CALORIE IS THE AMOUNT OF HEAT REQUIRED TO RAISE THE TEMPERATURE OF ONE LITRE OF WATER THROUGH 1 DEGREE CENTRIGRADE. IT IS KNOWN AS K.cal.

- 1 gram of carbohydrate = 4 k.cal
- 1 gram of fat = 9 k.cal
- 1 gram of protein = 4 k.cal

Body Building Function

Proper kind and amount of food, if taken, can assure us of body growth and development. A new born baby of 2.7 to 3.2 kg can grow upto 50.60 kg. If he takes right kind and amount of food from birth to adulthood. The food eaten each day helps to maintain the structure of the adult body, and to replace worn out cell of the body.

Although all the nutrients help in this function, the major nutrients are proteins, minerals, and water. Water is one of the main component of each cell body and it forms about 65 percent of our total body weight. Protein are main building block of every cell.

Regulation of the Body Process

In our body various process keeps going on and food helps in regulation of those process. Apart from these, food also helps in protecting our body from various infections and diseases.

A number of reactions goes in our body with the help of enzymes such as pepsin, rennin, trypsin. All the enzymes are protein. Thus we can say that these protein helps in regulation of various process in our body, such as muscle contraction, blood clotting, water balance, etc. it also improve our body's resistance to disease. The vitamins keep our body and skin healthy and keep us away from disease.

PSYCHOLOGICAL FUNCTION

Food not only provide us various nutrients, but it also satisfies our hunger needs. Food must satisfy certain emotional needs. These includes a sense of security, love and affection.

Sharing of food is a token of friendship and acceptance.

Food cooked by our loved one adds to joy of eating. This is known as psychological aspect of food which gives us psychological satisfaction.

SOCIAL FUNCTION

FOOD has always been a central part of our social existence. Food creates an atmosphere where the social relations can be developed and it helps in bringing the people from different class and communities.

Food has been used as an expression of love, friendship, and social acceptance. It is also used as a symbol of happiness at certain events in life. For example, laddus are associated with the celebration of Deewali, a marriage as cakes are associated with birthday, and Christmas.

chapter thirty-seven

Macronutrients and their Functions

The macronutrients are those nutrients which are present in larger amount in any food group. For example rice, which has 78.2 gram percent carbohydrate, 6.9 gram of proteins and 0.5 gram of fat.

Micronutrients are those nutrient which are present in very small amount in any food group, as in rice. 06 mg percent of vitaminB, 10 mg of calcium.

Thus the nutrients are divided into two categories.

Macronutrients—Carbohydrates, fat, protein, water.

Micronutrients—Vitamins, minerals.

MARCONUTRIENTS

Carbohydrates

These are simple sugar or polymers of sugar such as starch that can be hydrolyzed to simple sugar by the action of digestive enzyme. They contain carbon, hydrogen, and oxygen hence, called as carbohydrate. Carbohydrate is the nutrient that we consume daily in the maximum amount. These are either naturally present in rice, wheat, fruits, honey, potato, or added to food in the form of sugar.

Function of Carbohydrates

- Energy giving action—The primary function of carbohydrates in the body is to supply energy. Each gram of carbohydrate provides 4 kcal energy to the body. Which is needed for physical activities.
- Carbohydrates also act as reserve fuel supply in the form of glycogen stored in muscle and liver. The total amount of glycogen in the body is over 300 gram, but it must be mentained by regular intake of carbohydrates at frequent intervals, so that the breakdown of fat and protein tissue is prevented.
- Regulation of fat metabolism—Carbohydrate when present in adequate amount in the diet, helps in the proper utilisation of the fat in the body.
- Carbohydrates and their derivatives work as precursors of important metabolic compound. These includes nucleic acid, the matrix of connective tissues, and galactosides of nerve tissue.
- Lactose, the milk sugar, provides galactose, needed for brain development. It aids absorption of calcium and phosphorus, thus helping bone growth and maintenance.
- It helps to increase our resistance to infection.

- Carbohydrates are needed to prevent dehydration. A low carbohydrate diet causes loss of water from tissues as electrolytes, in the urine and can lead to involuntary dehydration.
- Fiber and roughage present in diet which are not digested by the body, provides bulk to the diet and helps in the normal movement of the food in the gastro-intestinal tract. This helps to prevent constipation. These are present in green leafy vegetables, fruits.

  Carbohydrate like sugar, honey and jaggery enhances flavor of the food and helps to make tasty.

Food Sources Rich in Carbohydrates

Rice, rawa, wheat flour, banana, potato, chiku, mango, sugar, milk, beetroot, cake, icecream.

Recommended Dietary Allowance

Minimum 100 gram of carbohydrate are needed in the diet to ensure the efficient oxidation of fat. If the carbohydrates are taken in excess amount, converted in to fat and is reserved in body. As it is the cheapest source of food, which provides maximum amount of energy, it supplies up to 80 percent of the total calories.

Clinical Problems

- Low carbohydrate diet—Diet low in carbohydrate leads to ketosis which is characterised by excessive fatigue, dehydration, waterloss, and electrolyte deficits. Lack of carbohydrate in the diet basically causes lack of energy. This leads to underweight, tiredness and poor working efficiency.
- High carbohydrate diet—Nutritional adequacy—An excessive intake of sugar, candies, cakes, cookies, pastries, leads to overweight.
- Dental caries—Sugar provides the energy for bacterial growth, which leads to gradual build up of plaque, a sticky carbohydrate bacterial matrix that adheres firmly to the teeth and this gradually erode the tooth enamel and forms decay.
- Sugar and chronic disease—High carbohydrate diet, do not cause diabetes, but it may aggravate the condition.

Fat

Fats are most concentrated source of energy. They form an important part of our daily food. The cell and tissues of our body have fat as an integral part. The vital organs are protected by a sheath of fat and water, which prevents them from any injury.

Function of Fat

- Fats are the richest source of energy, one gram of fat gives 9 kcal, which is more than double the amount obtained from equal amount of carbohydrate and protein.
- Fat soluble vitamins like A, D, E and K, need fat for their proper absorption and utilisation in the body.

- The fat layer under the skin helps in maintaining body temperature.
- Fat acts as cushion for important organs in body and protects them from shocks and external injury.
- Fats are used for cooking and frying and make the food tasty and acceptable.
- They take longer time to be digested in the body. This gives us a feeling of fullness and satisfaction.

Fats are used to synthesise phospholipids which are found in all cell.

Food sources: Vegetable oil which is extracted from oil seeds and nuts such as ground nut, mustard, sesame, soyabean, coconut, cottonseed. Butter and *ghee* are animal fat, extracted from milk. The animal food, milk, liver, meat, egg which contains fat are sources of hidden fat in the diet. They also supply protein, minerals, and vitamin B. *Ghee*, butter, liver are good sources of vitamin A.

Recommended Dietary Allowances

About 10 percent of the total energy need is met by invisible fat in the diet, 5 percent of the total energy should be provided by visible fat. 12 gram of fat per day fulfil this requirement for a normal adult.

Clinical Problems

- Deficiency of fat—Fat has an effect on body whether they are less or excess in diet lack of fat in diet basically causes lack of energy. This leads to underweight, tiredness, and reduced working efficiency. The body can suffer from deficiency of vitamin A, D, E, and K. If enough fat is not present in the diet.
- Excess of fat—Certain amount of fat is essential for our health, but excess of it can lead to ill health. Excess amount of fat leads to obesity and unacceptable blood lipid profile. This further leads to deposition of fatty material with formation of plaques in the arteries, which disturbs the movement of oxygen and nutrients, which further leads to variety of heart ailments, such as atherosclerosis, and high blood pressure.

Proteins

Protein is the chief component of all body tissue. Protein is now retained as a group name to designate the principal nitrogenous constituents of the protoplasm of all living tissues, and for innumerable regulatory function.

Function of Protein

- Maintenance and growth—Protein constitute the chief solid matter of muscle, organ and endocrine glands. They are major constituents of the matrix, of bone and teeth, skin, nails and hair, and blood cell, and serum. Our body which consists of about 60 percent water, and 19 percent fat, 17 percent of protein and 4 percent minerals.

- Regulation of body process—Body proteins have highly specialised function in the regulation of body process.
  - Nucleo protein contains the blue print for the synthesis of all body proteins.
  - Catalytic protein, the enzymes, number in thousand to facilitate each step of digestion, absorption, anabolism, and catabolism.
  - Hormonal protein set or release the brakes that control metabolic process.
  - Immune protein maintain the body's resistance to disease.
  - Contractile protein (myosin, actin) regulates muscle contraction.
  - Blood protein includes, a wide variety of function. The transport protein ferry nutrients to the tissues, for example hemoglobin, lipoproteins, transferrin (iron transport), retinol (binding protein), vitamin A (transport) and others. Hemoglobin is involved not only in transport of oxygen and carbon dioxide but contributes to acid- base balance. The serum protein, especially serum albumin which regulates osmotic pressure and maintains the fluid balance.

Tryptophan acts as a precursor for niacin and also for serotonin, a vasoconstrictor, methionine supplies labile methyl groups for the synthesis of choline, which helps to prevent storage of fat in the liver, glycine contributes to the formation of the porphyrin ring in the hemoglobin molecule and is also an important constituent of the purines and pyrimidines in nucleic acid.

- Energy—Proteins are a potential source of energy, each gram of protein gives 4 k.cal. If the diet is not proper to fulfil the demand from carbohydrate and fat, protein will be catabolised for energy.
- Histidine is used in the synthesis of histamine used as a vaso-dilator in the circulatory system. Glutamic acid is a precursor of a neurotransmitter. Phenylalanine is a precursor of tyrosine and together they lead to the formation of thyroxine and epinephrine. Tyrosin is also the precursor of skin and hair pigment.
- Milk formation—Human milk contains 1.2 percent protein. The milk proteins are synthesised in the mammary gland from the available dietary and tissue proteins. A nursing mother needs to take extra protein in the diet to meat the demands of protein for milk formation.

Food Sources

- Animal protein sources—Milk, egg, meat, fish, poultry and milk products like –cheese, curd, *khoa*. Salted or smoked fish and meat are very good source of proteins.
- Vegetable protein sources—Pulses like whole and split soyabeans, nuts, and oilseeds like peanut, almonds and cashewnut are rich source of vegetable protein. Cereals like wheat and rice also provide some amount of protein, dry beans, peas, dal when combined with small amount of egg, cheese, meat, fish and poultry provides satisfactory biological need.

Recommended Dietary Allowances

The requirement of the body for protein is determined by nitrogen balance studies, is between 0.5 to 0.6 gram per kg. Of body weight in adults, when the source of protein supplies the amino acid in the proportion needed by the body. In practice, the amino acid of the food combination may not be in so well proportion, therefore the recommended daily allowance for protein is set to 1.0 gram/kg of body weight for adult.

During infancy, pregnancy and lactation there is an increased need for protein. Person suffering from burns, tuberculosis, and rheumatic fever, also need additional protein for regeneration of wasted tissue.

FACTOR AFFECTING THE PROTEIN REQUIREMENT

- Sufficient protein for adult is needed to cover daily nitrogen losses in the urine, feces, desquamated skin, hair, nails, perspiration, and other secretions.
- Essential amino acid must be present in sufficient amount to meet the daily needs for tissue regeneration.
- Sufficient calories must be furnished to meet energy needs so that protein is not often used for energy. Thus, carbohydrates are fat 'spare' protein for its synthetic function.
- Growth, need of infants and children increases the protein requirement per kilogram of body weight.
- Development of material tissue and the fetus during pregnancy increases the protein need.
- Milk production by the mother increases the protein need.
- Infection, immobilisation, surgery, burns and other injuries increases protein catabolism and hence, the protein requirement.
- Emotional stress increases protein catabolism.
- Diseases of malabsorption can seriously interfere with digestion and absorption, thus increasing the demand for protein.

CLINICAL PROBLEM

- *Excess of proteins:* Protein is a vital need of the body, excess intake of protein gives stress on the body function. The liver has to demonise the extra amino acid and synthesise urea. The loss of calcium in the urine is increased with high protein intake. High protein from animal food carries undesirable saturated fats also along with it.
- *Protein deficiency:* Latent stage- the deficiency of protein accompanied by that of energy is one of the most common nutritional deficiencies.

  Children tend to have retarded growth. Protein deficiency during pregnancy may result in stress, which can lead to vomiting, swelling of feet. It may adversely affect the growth of the fetus and fetal stores for future. Thus, the infant's survival and health are affected by maternal nutrition. In children, lack of protein in the diet result in stunted growth and low weight.
- *Severe deficiency*—If there is severe deficiency of protein in the first two years of life, it could affect mental development, learning ability and behavior.
- *Kwashiorkar*—Occurs in children shortly after weaning, usually between the age of 1 to 4 years and it is characterised by growth failure, skin lesions, edema, and change in hair colour. The liver is extensively infiltrated with fat.

- *Marasmus*—It is usually seen earlier than kwashiorkor and is caused by a deficiency of both protein and calories. Growth failure is even more severe than in kwashiorkor but edema is usually absent.
- *Water*—Water is the most abundantly found nutrient in our body. It constitutes about 2/3 of our total body weight. It is present in every cell of the body and its basic functions are that of giving structure to the cell and participating in metabolic activities.

Water is important to maintain our body temperature. It also acts as a medium in which the body substances can dissolve and thus be transported and used in the body. It is also the main component of urine formed in the body, thus helping in the excretion of waste material from the body. As the water surrounds the internal body tissues, it protects them from external shocks and injuries. We should take Plenty of water as such or in the form of juices, milk and beverages like, tea.

chapter thirty-eight

Micronutrients

VITAMINS

Vitamins are nutrients which are very important for good health. They are required in small amounts, our body cannot synthesise them on its own; therefore, they must be provided by food. The lack of vitamins in the diet leads to various deficiency diseases. They are divided into two groups, on the basis of their solubility into fat soluble and water soluble vitamins fat soluble vitamin include A, D, E and K, water soluble vitamins include the B-complex, and vitamin C.

FAT-SOLUBLE VITAMIN

This was the first fat-soluble vitamin to be discovered. It has a number of important functions in the body. It is active in many forms.

Retinol—Vitamin A.

Retinylesters—Vitamin A esters.

Retinaldehyde—Vitamin A aldehyde, Retinal, Retinene.

Retinoic Acid—Vitamin A acid.

The chief source in human nutrition is beta—Carotene, which the body converts to Vitamin A in the intestinal mucosa during absorption. The conversion is partial and varies from 25 to 50 %.

Measurement—Vitamin A is measured in international unit the equivalents are

ITU—0.3 ug retinol.

ITU—0.6 ug beta-carotene.

ITU—1.2 ug other proVitamin A carotenoids.

Function

Vitamin A has various functions in the body. It is necessary for normal growth and development. If the intake of Vitamin A is not sufficient for normal growth, the bones stop its normal growth. Some time it may results in degeneration of nervous tissue without causing bone malformation.

a. Vision—The best understood function of Vitamin A is related to the maintenance of normal vision in dimlight. The retina of eye contains two kinds of light receptors, the rods for vision in dimlight and the cones for vision in bright light and colour vision. The rods produce a photosensitive pigment, Rhodopsin or visual purple, and the cones produce Iodopsin or visual violet.

In both these Pigments Vitamin A in the form of retinaldehyde is the prosthetic group, but the proteins to which the aldehyde is attached are different. When light strikes the Pigments, changes occur in the chemical configuration of retinaldehydes and the Pigments are split into their component part, Retinaldehyde and protein. These changes initiate a nerve impulse that is then transmitted to the brain by way of the optic nerve. Regeneration of rhodopsin occurs in the dark, but some retinaldehyde is lost in each cycle so that a constant supply from the blood must be present.

b. Health of epithelial tissues—Vitamin A is required for healthy epithelium whether covering the body externally or lining the mucous membranes. If affects the synthesis of constituents of mucus such as the mucoproteins and the mucopolysaccharides. The mucous secretion maintains the integrity of the epithelium, especially the membranes that line the eyes, the mouth, and the gastrointestinal, respiratory and genitourinary tracts. These membranes maintained in their optimum condition offer resistance to bacterial invasion, to that extent Vitamin A gives protection against infection.

c. Haemopoesis—Vitamin A deficiency in man is consistently associated with an iron deficiency anemia. In these conditions, Vitamin A is required in addition to iron for a full response.

d. Growth—Vitamin A is essential for normal skeletal and tooth development.

e. Energy Balance—Mitochondrial enzymes, which controls the local production of energy as heat is under the transcriptional regulation of Retinoic acid.

f. Vitamin A is essential for spermatogenesis in the male and normal estrus cycle in female.

g. The Synthesis of hydrocholesterol is facilitated in the adrenal cortex by Vitamin A.

h. Vitamin A also influences Synthesis of both serum and muscle proteins and its apparent effect on cell differentiation is related to a role in DNA and RNA metabolism.

Food sources—Only animal food contains Vitamin A.

Milk, Butter, Cheese, liver and egg yolk contains Vitamin A. Liver is the richest source of Vitamin A.

The Principal source of Vitamin A in the diet is from Carotenes, which are found in dark green or yellow food.

Green Leafy Vegetables—Spinach, drum stick, leaves cabbage, beet greens, broccoli, palak. Yellow fruits like Mango, Papaya, Carrot, sweat Potatoes, Pumpkin, Apricot Orange.

Recommended Daily Allowance

The daily requirement of an adult for Vitamin A is 600 mcg of retinol or 2400 mcg of beta-carotene per day derived from foods of either animal or vegetable.

For Infants 350 mcg. The need gradually increases as the child grows. During pregnancy there is no change in RDA but it is increased to 950 mcg or 3800 mcg of beta-carotene during lactation.

Clinical Problems

Deficiency of Vitamin A

a. Night blindness—Night blindness or NYCTALOPIA is a condition in which the individual is unable to see well in dim light, especially on coming into darkness from a bright light.

NYCTALOPIA occurs when there is insufficient Vitamin A to bring about prompt and complete regeneration of visual purple.

Next symptoms is usually dryness of lining of eyelids and eyeball (conjunctiva). A later arid more severe stage of deficiency is xerosis of the cornea. The cornea becomes dry and loses its transparency (xerophthalmia). In the last stage of keratomalacia, the cornea becomes soft and results in permanent blindness.

b. Epithelial changes—An inadequate supply of Vitamin A may lead to definite changes in the epithelial tissues throughout the body KERATIZATION. It is characterised by shrinking, hardening and progressive degeneration of the cells. Skin changes in severe Vitamin A deficiency known as Follicular Hyperkeratosis. The skin becomes rough, dry and scaly.

Excess of Vitamin A

Excessive intake of Vitamin A are toxic to both children and adult. The common symptoms of toxicity are anorexia, hyperirritability, and drying and desquamation of the skin. Loss of hair, bone and joint pain, headache, enlargement of liver and spleen.

Vitamin D

Pure Vitamin D was isolated in Crystalline form in 1930 and was called calciferol. Vitamin D is also called "Sunshine Vitamin" because the body is able to convert a precursor 7—dehydrocholesterol, a sterol present in the skin, to Vitamin D in the presence of sunlight.

Vitamin D activity is shown by a group of chemical substances called sterols, which are wax like substance. These compounds are insoluble in water, but are soluble in fats. They are stable to acids, alkalies and heat.

Function

Calcitriol, activated form of Vitamin D, helps in absorption of calcium and Phosphorus. It acts with two other hormones Parathyroid and thyroid hormone calcitonin, and stimulates the absorption of calcium and phosphorus in the small intestine. Vitamin D helps in the formation of strong bone.

Recommended dietary allowance—100 IU is sufficient for bone development and prevent rickets for full term or premature infant 400 IU is recommended. 400 IU (10ug) is recommended daily for children and adolescents through 18 years of age. The allowance is reduced to 300 IU during the age of 10 to 22 years. Further reduce to 200 IU after the age of 22 years.

Food sources—Richest known source is fish liver oil Fortified foods, apart from this Irradiation of the body with sunlight is the main source of Vitamin D. The mid day sun is rich in Ultra-violet light and helps in synthesising Vitamin D.

Clinical Problems

Vitamin D Deficiency—Vitamin D deficiency leads to inadequate absorption of calcium and phosphorus from the intestinal tract and leads to faulty mineralization of bone and tooth structure. It also results to skeletal malformation.

Rickets—Improper supplement to Vitamin D leads to Rickets, where delayed closure of the fontanelles, softening of the skull, and bulging of the forehead, which gives head a boxlike appearance. It is further characterised by soft, fragile bone, enlargement of wrist, knee (knonk knee) and ankle joint, lack of muscle tone, pot belly.

Osteomalacia—It can be also referred as 'adult Rickets' which is characterised by softening of bone, pain general weakness, spontaneous multiple fractures, it occurs due to lack of Vitamin D and calcium.

Excess of Vitamin D—Excess of Vitamin D leads to toxicity which is characterised by nausea, diarrhoea, vomiting, weight loss, and polyuria. In severe cases, it may lead to renal damage calcification of soft tissues such as heart, blood vessels, bronchi, stomach.

Vitamin K

Dr. Dam found it in 1935 as a 'coagulation vitamin'. Which promotes normal blood clotting.

Function—Vitamin K is essential for the formation of PROTHROMBIN and other clotting proteins by the liver, which helps in blood clotting process.

Food sources—Green leafy vegetables such as Spinach, Cabbage, Cauliflower, Methi, Radish leaves.

Daily allowances—The Indian RDA committee considered that no recommended need made for Vitamin K. It is suggested that 0.5 to 1.0 mg of Vitamin K should be sufficient.

Clinical problems—A low blood of Prothrombin and other clotting factors leads to increased tendency to hemorrhage.

Deficiency may occur in adults because of a failure in absorption, on interference in synthesis in the intestine or inability to form Prothrombin by the liver.

Vitamin E

This is also a fat-soluble vitamin.

Function—It reduces oxidation of Vitamin A, Carotenes and polyunsaturated fatty acids. Selenium is a trace mineral that works as a partner with Vitamin E as an antioxident.

Food sources—Plant tissue, vegetable oils, wheat germ, rice germ, green leafy vegetables, nuts, legumes, coconut, soyabean.

Daily allowances
Infant—3-4 mg
Men—10 mg
Women—8 mg
Lactation—11 mg

Clinical problems—Deficiency leads to increased hemolysis of red blood cells, creatinuria, deposition of brownish ceroid pigment in smooth muscle. Vitamin E deficiency may lead to cystic fibrosis in small children.

WATER SOLUBLE VITAMIN

Water soluble vitamins consist of a large number of substances. The water-soluble vitamins are absorbed quickly in the body and amounts which is not utilized excreted in the urine therefore, sufficient amount should be given in daily diet.

Vitamin B-complex

These are a group of vitamins which are present in some food. They are thiamin, riboflavin, niacin, pyridoxine, folic acid and Vitamin B12.

Thiamin (Vitamin B1)

Function—The basic function of thiamin as a coenzyme is related to release of energy from glucose and its storage as fat, thus it makes energy available for normal growth and function of the body, Thiamin Pyrophosphate, the Coenzyme form of thiamin, is necessary for catalysing the oxidation of Carbohydrates in the body. This reaction release energy in the system.

Food sources
All unprocessed food contains Vitamin B1.
Nuts, lentils, Oat, Soyabean, Pork, Whole grain Wheat, Almond, Egg yolk, Liver, Peas are good sources of Vitamin B1.

Recommended daily allowance—The amount of thiamin requirement is Proportional to the calorie requirement. The minimum requirement is about 0.33 to 0.35 mg per 1,000 kcal. And RDA is 0.5 mg per 1,000kcal.

Clinical Problems

Deficiency—Lack of Vitamin B1 in and adult causes loss of appetite, nausea, loss of weight and weakness followed by polyneuritis with numbness and muscular paralysis. In the young there is almost complete stoppage of growth and death can be rapid. This condition is known as Beri-Beri.

Thiamin deficiency also leads to enlargement of the heart, tachycardia, and palpitation on exertion.

Riboflavin (Vitamin B2)

Riboflavin is very stable to heat, acid and air but it gets destroy in sunlight (Ultra-violet light). The name Riboflavin is derived from its chemical structure. It is yellow-green fluorescent pigment containing the sugar 'Ribose' so it's called Riboflavin.

Function—Vitamin B2 is present in all the cells of the body, where it forms part of several enzymes involved in the release of energy during the metabolism of glucose and fatty acids. It is also involved, with Vitamin B6, in the conversion of the amino acid tryptophan to the vitamin niacin. Vitamin B2 also acts in the conversion of folate to its active forms and as these are necessary for the synthesis of DNA, Vitamin B2 is involved in tissue growth and cell reproduction.

Food sources—Milk is the Rich source of Riboflavin, Milk products like, Cheese, Curd, Butter, Almond, Egg, Liver, Beans, Lenthil, Mushrooms, Soyabean, Spinach.

Recommended Daily Allowance
Men—1.6 mg
Women—1.2 mg
Pregnancy— + 0.3 mg
Lactation— + 0.5 mg
Children under 11—0.8-1.4 mg
Boys and girls—1.3-1.7 mg

Clinical problems—Deficiency causes Cheilosis (cracks at corners of lips). Scaly desuamation around Nose, Ear, Burning and Itching of Eye, Photo phobia.

Niacin

Niacin includes both nicotinic acid and nicotinamide is an other vitamin of vitamin B-complex group. It is highly soluble in water. Both components are stable and are not affected by heat, acid or alkali.

Function—Niacin acts as a component of two enzymes NAD and NADP. These enzymes are involved in tissue respiration and synthesis and the breakdown of glucose of product energy.

Food sources—Meat, Poultry, Fish, Whole grain and Whole wheat bread, Flours, Cereals, Nuts, Legumes, Bajra, Jowar, Potato, Liver.

Recommended daily allowances—Niacin is involved in the Utilisation of Carbohydrates, the requirement of niacin is related to the total Calories in the diet.
Men—18 mg
Women—13 mg
Pregnancy— + 2 mg
Lactation— + 5 mg
Boys and girls—14-19 mg
Infant—6-8 mg

Clinical problems—Lack of niacin affects the skin, gastrointestinal tract and nervous system. Causes anorexia, glossitis, diarrhoea, dermatitis, neurological degeneration. The deficiency disease is known as Pellagra which is seen in endemic form in some parts of India, where Jowar is the staple food.

Folic Acid

Folic acid and related compounds, which is one of the Vitamins B. It's name was derived from the Latin word folium, which means, leaf because it was first isolated from spinach leaves and is widely distributed in green leafy plants.

Folic acid is Pteroyl-mono-glutanic acid. It is quite soluble in slightly alkaline or acid solution but it is stable in neutral or alkaline solution, especially in the absence of air.

Function—Active form is folinic acid, requires ascorbic acid for conversion, coenzyme for transmethylation, synthesis of nucleoproteins; maturation of red blood cells, inter related with vitamin B-12. Folic acid undergoes a series of metabolic conversions to its various co-enzyme forms after it is absorbed.

Food sources—Green leafy vegetables, Liver, Legumes, poultry, Fish, Whole grain cereals are good source of folic acid.

Daily recommended allowances
Adults—400 ug
Pregnancy—800 ug
Lactation—500 ug
Infants—30-45 ug
Boys and girls—400 ug

Vitamin B12

Vitamin B12 contains, cobalt and phosphorus and is red in colour.
Vitamin B12 considered the most potent vitamin, but it is present in the body only in small amount.

They are slightly soluble in water, stable to heat, but are inactivated by light and by strong acid or alkaline solutions.

Function—It promotes normal growth and development. It helps with certain type of nerve damage, and treats pernicious anemia. In Bone Marrow B-12 coenzyme participates in the synthesis of DNA. It is essential for the normal functioning of all cells, especially of bone marrow, the nervous system and gastrointestinal tract.

Food sources—There is no Vitamin B12 in Plants. The richest sources are organ meat, milk, egg, and fish.

It is not stable to heat and light.

Recommended daily allowances
Adults—3 ug
Pregnancy—4 ug
Lactation—4 ug
Infant—0.5-1.5 ug
Boys & girls—3 ug.

Clinical problems—Lack of intrinsic factor leads to deficiency, pernicious anemia, following gastrectomy, macrocytic anemia or megaloblast anemia.

In the nervous system, lack of B12 causes severe degeneration of the spinal cord, due partly to inadequate production of the myelin sheath around the long fibres.

Vitamin C

It is also known as Ascorbic Acid. It is easily destroyed on exposure to heat and light. The vitamin is a while, crystalline, odourless compound, soluble in water.

Function—It plays a very important role to build and maintain strong tissues especially connective tissues (Bone, Cartilage, Collagen). Blood Vessel tissue depends on Vitamin C to form strong capillary walls.

It helps in Synthesis of Collagen, Absorption and use of iron. It helps the body to build resistance to infection. It helps in the absorption of calcium and strengthens the bone. It is needed in wound healing infections to help recovery.

Food sources—Citrus fruits, Amla, Tomatoes, Melons, Guava, Papaya, Pineapple, Drumstick leaves, Capsicum, Cashew fruits are main source of Vitamin C.

Recommended daily allowances
Men—60 mg
Women—60 mg
Pregnancy—80 mg
Lactation—100 mg
Infant—35 mg
Boys and girls—50 mg.

Clinical problems—Vitamin C deficiency weakened Cartilage and Capillary walls, Cutaneous hemorrhages, Causes bleeding gums, Poor wound healing, Poor bone and tooth development, scurvy.

Minerals

Mineral are those elements that remain largely as ash when plant or animal tissues are burned. About 4 % of the body weight consist of mineral matter. Calcium and phosphorus accounts for ¾ of all minerals in our body. They are present in all body tissues and fluids.

Mineral does not destroy during food preparation and also it do not provide energy.

Calcium

Compared to other minerals, calcium is present in larger quantity in our body. It is present in almost every cell of the body. But the maximum amount is present in bones, and teeth along with phosphorus. These give the skeleton structure and rigidity.

Function

1. It is involved in normal muscle contraction, which include heart beat.
2. It helps in maintenance of permeability of cell membranes to permit movement of material in and out of the cells.
3. Helps in normal clotting of blood.
4. Activates action of enzymes.
5. Ensure the absorption of Vitamin B12.

Food sources—Milk is the richest source of Calcium, Cheese, Paneer, Mava, SMP are good.

Sources of calcium—Ragi and seasame seeds have high concentration of calcium. Dark green leafy vegetable are a good source of calcium.

Recommended daily allowances
Adults—800 mg
Children 1 to 10 years—1,200 mg
Pregnant and Lactating Women—360 to 540 mg.

Clinical Problems
Osteomalacia is a reduction in the mineral content of the bone without reduction in bone size.
Osteoporosis is a reduction in the total bone mass. This is found more in women than man.

When a pregnant women does not get proper amount of calcium lose calcium from their body tissues to supply the needs of the fetus.

In children lack of calcium affects their growth. The skeletal frame does not mineralise properly, resulting in weak bone. The teeth are also affected.

Tetany is a condition characterised by a low blood calcium, increased excitability of the nerves, and uncontrolled contractions of the muscles.

Hypercalcemis—Milk-alkali syndrome in which patients with peptic ulcer have used excessive amount of readily absorbed alkalies together with large amount of milk over a period of years. This is characterised by vomiting, increases in blood pressure, gastrointestinal bleeding.

Phosphorus—Phosphorus contains about 1 % of boy weight or ¼ of the total mineral matter in the body.

Function
1. Phosphorus is a constituent of the sugar—phosphate linkage in the structures of DNA and RNA, the substances that controls heredity.
2. As a part of ATP and ADP which are essential for energy metabolism in the body.
3. Phospholipids are constituents of cell membranes, thus regulates the transport of solutes.
4. Inorganic phosphates in the body fluids constitute an important buffer system in the regulation of body neutrality.

Food sources—Milk, Egg, Flesh foods, Legumes and Nuts are good sources of Phosphorus.

Recommended daily allowances—Same as calcium, except for infants.
During first 6 months of life—240 mg

Magnesium

The amount of magnesium in the body is much smaller than calcium and phosphorus. Bones and teeth contains 60 percent of magnesium.

Function—Magnesium acts like a Catalyst in various metabolic reaction. It is also involved in protein synthesis. It regulates muscle contraction, regulates transmission of nerve stimuli.

Food sources—Dark green leafy vegetables are good source of Magnesium.

Recommended daily allowances
Men—350 mg
Women—300 mg.
Pregnancy and Lactation—450 mg

Clinical problems—Deficiency is characterised by muscle tremor, paresthesias and convulsive seizures and delirium.

TRACE ELEMENTS

Iron

Another important mineral for the body is Iron. It is required in very small amount by the body and is therefore, also called as Trace element.

Function

1. Iron combines with protein for the development of hemoglobin, the red pigment of the blood. It acts as a carrier of oxygen from the lungs to the tissues and indirectly helps in the return of Carbon dioxide to the lungs.
2. Myoglobin is an iron-protein present in muscle which store some oxygen for immediate use by the cell.

Food sources—Eggs, Liver and Meat contains iron in a readily available form. Leafy vegetables, Cereals such as Whole Wheat Flour, rice millet, Pulses, Bajra, Ragi Jowar are also good sources of iron.

Daily recommended allowances
Men and non Menstruating women—10 mg
Menstruating Women—18 mg
Pregnant Women—18 + mg
Children—10-15 mg
Infants—10-15 mg

Clinical problems—Iron-Deficiency Anemia. The lack of iron result in anemia due to insufficiency of hemoglobin. Person lacking iron get tired easily, feet & faint due to inability of the body to carry sufficient oxygen to the cells for respiration.

Hemosiderosis is a disorder of iron metabolism in which large amount of iron is absorbed and deposited in the Liver, Lungs, Pancreas.

Hemochromatosis is a genetic defect, in which there is excessive absorption of iron resulting in organ damage and skin pigmentation. It may lead to cirrhosis of liver.

Iodine

About 1/3 of the iodine in the adult is found in the thyroid gland where it is stored in the form of Thyroglobulin. Two hormones produced by the thyroid—Triiodothyroxine (T3) and Thyroxine (T4) contain iodine. These hormones monitor the rate of energy. Metabolism in the body and thus are essential for growth and development.

Food sources—The most important source of iodine is iodized salt, seaweed, salt-water fish are also good source of iodine.

Daily recommended allowances
Men and women over the age of 11—150 ug
Infant—40 to 50 ug
Children upto 10 years—70 to 120 ug.

Clinical problems—Goiter is iodine deficiency disease characterised by an increase in the size and number of epithelial cells in the thyroid gland. Cretinism occurs in infant and is characterised by a low basal metabolism; muscular flabbiness and weakness dry skin, enlarged tongue, thick lips arrest skeletal development and severe mental retardation.

OTHER TRACE ELEMENTS

Apart from iodine and iron there are number of trace element required by the body as Copper, Zinc, Selenium, Cobalt, Fluorine, and Manganese.

chapter thirty-nine

Diet and Exercise

All the energy needed for growth and repair of the body, for muscular activity and for all the work done by cells comes from the metabolism of fat, carbohydrate, protein.

The amount of energy used during exercise is related movement. Frequent movement in body demands more energy, especially if the body is lifted rather than move horizontally.

Selection of an Exercise Programme

The choice of an exercise programme varies from person to person.
1. Choose an exercise, which you like to do.
2. Choose an exercise, which can be done in all seasons.
3. Choose an exercise for which you have the facilities and according to convenience.
4. Choose an exercise, which you can do regularly.
5. Choose an exercise, which involves your whole body.
6. Choose exercise according to goals and objectives.

Beginning of an Exercise Programme

It is always important to begin an exercise programme with a proper plan. Strong motivation and interest is necessary to start an exercise programme on a long-term basis. Some of the basic guidelines for the beginners are
1. Consult your Doctor.
2. Measure your weight, height, chest, waist and muscle girth, blood pressure joint function before starting any exercise programme.
3. Start of with warm-up exercises, followed by some basic stretching exercises.
4. Gradually increases the duration and intensity of an exercise. Initially 3 to 5 minutes should be sufficient for a sedentary person or old person.
5. Aerobic exercises are the best way to increase Physical fitness but, before starting, consult your doctor; they may help you to select the exercise programme according to your need.
6. Always finish your exercise session with cool down exercises.

Energy System Used by the Body

1. ATP—(Adenosine Triphosphate) is the immediately usable form of chemical energy. Which is stored in muscle cells and it is used for muscular activity. The ATP-PC system is an anaerobic energy system that resynthesises ATP from energy released when phosphocreatine (PC) is broken. It is very rapid but limited source of ATP that is used during high-power, short-duration activities.

Table 39.1

Sr. No.	Prescription	Effect
1	Warm-up Exercise (Major joints are moved through their range of motion.)	- Patient's first step/ checks how body feels before exercise. - Helps to increase joint Lubrication - Some Flexibility gain.
2.	Circulatory Warm-up (Ligh Aerobic Exercise)	- Increases tissue temperature and synovial fluid in preparation for stretching. - Gradual preparation for heart and circulatory system. - Stimulates joint Mechanics.
3.	Warm-up (Stretch, emphasis on Static Stretching) Warm-up continues in the activity to resistance	- Increases Flexibility - Target Muscle used, if used eccentrically. - Dynamic stretches for sports preparation. - With a light overload follow (start progressive)
4.	Aerobic Exercise (in a Progressive way)	- Build up gradually, whether continuous or in interval - Avoid final sprints or sudden stop - Heart rate increases. - Muscular tightness, if any is stretched.
5.	Sports	- Do a mini warm-up - Stretch Tight Muscle - Tend immediately to minor injury.
6.	Resistance Exercise	- Progressive Resistance & adequate interval (depends on treatment method. - Incorporate warm-up set.
7.	Muscle Balance	- Check the balance (agonist and antagonist muscle group i.e. there is a need for specific muscle stretch to strengthening) Checks for Muscular tightness, fatigue, inflammation, and minor injuries (modify the exercise around injury) correct breathing, pulse rate.
8.	Cool Down Exercise (Stretch, Static Stretching)	- Gives maximum flexibility - Specific Muscle used, if used eccentrically.

Before living have a self-check for heart rate, depth of Breathing, Muscle soreness or tightness, and any minor injuries. (If present ice should be kept over it.)

2. The lactic acid (LA) system—It is also an anaerobic, resynthesis ATP from energy released during the breakdown of glycogen to lactic acid. Accumulation of lactic acid causes muscular fatigue. This system is used mainly during activities that require between one and three minutes of maximum effort.

3. The oxygen system (O_2)—It utilises both glycogen and fat as fuel for ATP resynthesis. By a number of reactions that takes place in mitochondria, large amount of ATP is released. This aerobic system is used predominantly during endurance exercises.

REQUIREMENTS FOR MODERATE EXERCISE

Fluids and Oxygen

More water is needed with increase in exercise. All cellular activities take place in an aqueous medium. Water carries nutrients and waste products via blood stream to and from the cells. Thus sufficient blood volume should be there to ensure loss of heat produced through skin and sweat. Water is lost from the body through Sweat. Less fluid in the body may reduce sweating and blood flow, disturbing body temperature regulation. A water loss of 4 to 5 % reduces work capacity by 20 to 30 %. A 10 % loss may result in circulatory collapse.

The fluid loss in exercise depends on the duration and intensity of exercise as also the ambient temperature and humidity. Normal sweat production, without exercise is 500 to 700 ml per day. It may increase to 8 to 12 liters per day with prolonged exercises.

Electrolyte—Sweat contains electrolytes, such as chloride, magnesium, and potassium, performance is not disturbed by electrolyte losses. In hot places or hot season.

Dilute salt solution (1/2 teaspoon salt per liter) should be given during training.

During exercises, as heat is released with energy production, the body temperature rises. Sweat is an effort to control body temperature. The loss of water through sweat should be replaced to prevent dehydration.

Oxygen—The need for oxygen increases during exercise, as more oxygen is needed to release extra body energy. The ability of the body to provide the oxygen needed is known as aerobic capacity. The aerobic capacity is dependent on the fitness of tissues involved in oxygen intake and transport—lungs, heart and blood vessels and the body composition.

Nutritional needs for exercise—Any exercise activity increases energy production. Proper diet is an essential requirement for good performance. It is essential to have proper nutritional food to meet the demand during exercise. As we have seen before carbohydrates and fats are the basic suppliers of energy reserves, and protein gives very little energy.

Carbohydrates is the major nutrient to provide energy for exercise. Our body has two sources of carbohydrate reserves—the glucose in the circulating blood and the glycogen, stored in muscle and liver. For an active person, the diet needs to provide 55 to 60 % of total dietary calories in the form of complex Carbohydrates as they break down more slowly and helps to maintain blood sugar levels more evenly. Secondly, starches are more readily converted to glycogen to maintain this reserve store.

Fat—There is no need for increasing the level of fat in the diet. The total fat should not exceed 20 to 25 % of the total dietary calories.

Proteins—It is important to meet one's recommended dietary allowance (RDA) for protein. No additional protein is needed for exercise.

Vitamins and minerals—Any increase in metabolism increases the need for Vitamin B1, B2 and niacin. In general the efficient use of vitamins and minerals by the body is increased during exercise.

The athletes, who need more energy, take larger amount of nutritive food, which increases their intake of vitamins and minerals. Adolescent or female athletes may need extra iron supplements, if their blood iron level is very low.

BODY MASS INDEX

BMI is the widely accepted technique for weight assessment is developed by the National center for health statistics is called body mass index (BMI). BMI is calculated by measuring a person's weight in kilogram and dividing by that person's height in meter squared (kg/m) for example, an adult of 70 kg with a height of 1.75 meters has a BMI of 70 /1.75 =22.9 calculation of BMI is not difficult as it may seem. To get your kilogram weight, divide your weight in pounds (without shoes or clothing) by 2.2 to convert your height to meters squared, divide your height in inches (without shoes) by 39.4, then square this result.

Ideal body weight may also be defined as 100 percent to 119 percent and obese as > 120 percent of normal.

HYDROSTATIC WEIGHING TECHNIQUES

From a clinical perspective, the most accurate method of measuring body fat is through hydrostatic weighing technique. This method measures the amount of water a person displaces when completely submerged. Because fat tissue has a lower density than muscle or bone tissue, a relatively accurate indication of actual body fat can be calculated by comparing a person's under water and out-of-water weight.

PINCH AND SKINFOLD MEASURES

Most commonly used method of body fat measurement is pinch test studies shows the triceps area is one of the most reliable area of the body for assessing the fat in the subcutaneous layer of the skin.

A person pinches a fold of skin just behind the triceps with the thumb and the index finger if the size of the pinch appears to be thicker than 1 inch, the person is considered over fat.

Skin Fold Caliper Test

It is more accurate than pinch test in this method a person pinches skin folds at various points of the body with thumb and the index finger. This technique uses a caliper called skinfold caliper, which takes a precise measurement of fat layer. Accept triceps we should measure for biceps, subscapular area, and the iliac crest area.

Mid-arm(triceps) muscle circumference is measured using following equation.

Mid arm muscle circumference = mid upper arm circumference (in cm)—(π x triceps skin – fold thickness(in cm)

GIRTH AND CIRCUMFERENCE MEASURE

Another common method of body fat measurement is use of girth and circumference measure. Therapist use a measuring tape to take girth, circumference, measurement at various body parts. These measurements are then converted into constants, and a formula is used to determine relative percentage of body fat. Although this technique is inexpensive, easy to use, and commonly performed, it is not as accurate as other techniques.

SOFT-TISSUE ROENTGENOGRAM

This method involves injecting a radioactive substance into the body and allowing this substance to penetrate muscle(lean) tissue so distinctions between fat and lean tissue can be made by means of imaging.

BIOELECTRICAL IMPEDANCE ANALYSIS

BIA involves, sending a small electric current through the person's body. The amount of resistance to the current, along with the person's age, sex, and other physical characteristics, is then fed into a computer that uses special formula to determine the total amount of muscle and fat tissue.

TOTAL BODY ELECTRICAL CONDUCTIVITY

One of the recent assessment is total body electrical conductivity *(TOBEC)*, in this method therapist uses an electromagnetic force field to assess relative body fat.

Apart from these computed tomography,(CT) or magnetic resonance imaging (MRI), and electrical impedance.

General Bibliography

Acupuncture

1. Jayasuria Anton, Fernando Felix: *Principles and Practice of Scientific Acupuncture* (1st ed), 1978.
2. Mann Felix: *Acupuncture*, The Ancient Chinese Art of Healing and How it Works Scientifically (1st ed), 1973.
3. Needham J, L Gwei: Djen, Celestial Lancets, *A History and Rationale of Acupuncture and Moxa*, 1980.
4. Mann KF: *The Treatment of Disease By Acupuncture*, 1980 (3rd Ed).
5. Melzack R, Wall PD: *The Challenge of Pain*, 1982.
6. Kenyon, Dr. Julian: *Modern Techniques of Acupuncture*, 1986 (2nd Ed).
7. Stux, Dr. GB Pomeranz: *Basics of Acupuncture*, 1991 (2nd Ed).
8. Travell, JG DG Simons: *Myofascial Pain and Dysfunction the Triger Point Manual.*
9. Nightingale, Dr. Michael: *Healing Power of Acupuncture* (1st Ed).
10. Woo, Dr. Park Jae: Guide to Hand and Foot Acupuncture—1st Ed (1993).
11. Lee T-Sun Nin: *A Treatise on Acupuncture Meridians*, 1978.
12. Vaciavkajdos: *Theoretical Principles of Chinese Medicine*, 1973.

Yoga

1. Swami Satyananda Saraswati: *A Systemic Course in the Ancient Tantric Techniques of Yoga and Kriya.*
2. BKS Iyengar: *Light on Yoga.*
3. BKS Iyengar: *The Art of Yoga.*
4. BKS Iyengar: *Light on the Yoga Sutras of Patanjali.*
5. AC Guyton: *Textbook of Physiology.*
6. BD Chaurasia: *Human Anatomy.*
7. Rene Cailliet: *Low Back Pain Syndrome.*

Nutrition

1. Sumati R Mudambi, MV Rajagopal: *Fundamental of Foods And Nutrition.*
2. Rebecca J Donatelle, Lorraine G Davis: *Access to Health.*
3. Corinne H Robinson, Marilyn R Lawler: *Normal and Therapeutic Nutrition.*
4. HK Bakhru: *A Complete Handbook of Nature Cure.*
5. Brunner, Suddarth: *Medical Surgical Nursing.*
6. Wells Peter E: *Pain Management and Control in Physiotherapy.*

Index

READER SUGGESTIONS SHEET

Please help us to improve the quality of our publications by completing and returning this sheet to us.

Title/Author: **Alternative Therapies by Swati Bhagat PT**

Your name and address:

E-mail address,

Phone and Fax:

How did you hear about this book? [please tick appropriate box (es)]

☐ Direct mail from publisher   ☐ Conference   ☐ Bookshop

☐ Book review   ☐ Lecturer recommendation   ☐ Friends

☐ Other (please specify)   ☐ Website

Type of purchase: ☐ Direct purchase   ☐ Bookshop   ☐ Friends

Do you have any brief comments on the book?

Please return this sheet to the name and address given below.

JAYPEE BROTHERS
MEDICAL PUBLISHERS (P) LTD
EMCA House, 23/23B Ansari Road, Daryaganj
New Delhi 110 002, India

6-10-08 JP fd